EMERGENCY ENCOUNTERS

A STUDY OF AN URBAN AMBULANCE SERVICE

JAMES M. MANNON

National University Publications
KENNIKAT PRESS // 1981
Port Washington, N.Y. // London

Manufactured in the United States of America

Published by
Kennikat Press Corp.
Port Washington, N.Y. / London

Library of Congress Cataloging in Publication Data

Mannon, James M   1942–
    Emergency encounters.

    (Series in the sociology of medicine) (National university publications)
    Bibliography: p.
    Includes index.
    1. Ambulance service–United States–Case studies. 2. Emergency medical technicians–United States–Case studies. 3. Ambulance service–Sociological aspects. I. Title. II. Series.
RA995.5.A1M36   362.1'8'0973   80-26453
ISBN 0-8046-9281-5

CONTENTS

PREFACE

Emergency Encounters examines the social world of emergency ambulance work in one of the nation's largest cities. It is about the emergency medical technicians (EMTs) and paramedics who form the staff of a hospital-based ambulance service that responds to nearly 40,000 emergency calls per year. Although the book is mostly descriptive, it attempts to use a sociological perspective to gain greater understanding about the nature of emergency ambulance work. The focus is on decision making, teamwork, EMT/paramedic attitudes and values, aspects of professionalism, and the special stresses that accompany emergency work. None of the research that informs this book was gathered to test a specific theory, hypothesis, or model. The main purpose was to explore and describe how those men and women who earn their living doing emergency ambulance work come to terms with that work, cope with its hazards, and learn to derive some sense of satisfaction and reward from their occupation. Insofar as possible, I have tried to see and describe this world from the point of view of the EMT and paramedic: how they see themselves, their patients, and their work.

This study is based on data that was gathered through my own participant observation. In 1978 and 1979, I spent several hundred hours with the EMTs and paramedics at County Hospital—the research site. I rode in a variety of ambulances, accompanying the crews on their emergency runs. In my role as observer, I witnessed many emergency scenes in which the EMTs and paramedics attempted to be of help to patients. I visited many hospital emergency rooms and recorded the interactions between the ambulance crews and the emergency-room doctors and nurses. In addition, I spent many hours sitting in the various crew rooms listening to EMTs and paramedics talk to each other about their runs, their patients, and their colleagues. I asked numerous questions of the crews about what I had seen, and the answers I received helped to fill in the missing pieces that were needed to grasp the larger picture of ambulance work. One paramedic was gracious enough to give me in-depth answers to several key questions I had in regard to his work and career.

The book begins with a description of the setting, the background of the study, and the organization of an urban ambulance service. Chapter 2 focuses on the uncertainty inherent in emergency care, and how EMTs and paramedics attempt to reduce that uncertainty in making medical judgments and decisions. Chapter 3 is devoted to the special problems that must be faced in working as part of an emergency medical team. It analyzes how members of an ambulance crew develop interpersonal trust and learn to cooperate and accommodate with one another in order to create an effective partnership. Paramedics and EMTs must also learn to cooperate smoothly and effectively with other emergency workers, and the problematic aspects of their relationships with police, firemen, doctors and nurses, are addressed in Chapter 4. The values and attitudes of those who do emergency ambulance work are discussed in Chapter 5. The chapter describes what EMTs and paramedics like and dislike about their work—their moments of triumph and success, their tribulations and failures. Chapter 6 examines the professional future of the EMT and paramedic. Arguments are presented supporting the idea of emergency ambulance work as an emerging or nascent profession. Those who make their living responding to medical emergencies are daily exposed to a variety of strains, stresses, and risks; Chapter 7 describes the hardships that accompany the work of the EMT and paramedic; the phenomenon of burnout and its implications for careers in ambulance work are analyzed. Finally, the book concludes with my own reflections on my fieldwork experience. I explore my role as a participant observer of emergency ambulance crews.

A number of colleagues and friends provided me with encouragement while I was engaged in writing this book. Mike Rainey, my former teacher; Curt Bergstrand; Charles Flynn; and Rudy Seward were particularly supportive.

I would like to thank DePauw University for providing me with two faculty research grants which were generous enough to allow me to complete this work. Fred Silander, dean of the faculty, was especially encouraging in the early phases of the field research. I also would like to thank several of my students who were kind enough to read drafts of the manuscript and offer constructive comments: Lynn Fox, Cathy Miller, Leon Bell, and Mel Bedree.

Ruth Sargent, my typist, showed great patience and perseverance throughout the typing of several manuscript drafts. Her many kindnesses and words of encouragement meant much to me, and I now acknowledge my considerable debt to her.

I should like to thank everyone associated with Kennikat Press for their assistance in preparing this volume. An anonymous reviewer provided valuable criticism of an earlier draft which was quite helpful in making revisions.

My wife, Molly, and my daughters, Sarah and Susie, supported me during this entire undertaking. I have been only a part-time husband and father for three years now, and I thank them for not reminding me of this. Knowing that they cared so much about this project was a great help to me.

This study would not have been possible without the cooperation of the many administrators and EMTs and paramedics at the research site. Because of promises of anonymity, I am unable to identify by name the persons and institutions used in this research. But they themselves know who they are, and I sincerely thank them for all the help they gave me in so many ways. Those in top administrative positions in the ambulance division of County Hospital were helpful without exception, and it made my work considerably easier.

To the many EMTs and paramedics who are the subject of this research, I now record my deep appreciation. At all times, they showed much willingness to be scrutinized by an observer. To all those ambulance crews who allowed me to learn something about myself by learning about their work, I dedicate this book.

EMERGENCY ENCOUNTERS

ABOUT THE AUTHOR

James M. Mannon is an assistant professor of sociology at DePauw University in Greencastle, Indiana. He is the author of several articles in scholarly journals. He has recently served as a consultant to the Ambulance Division and the Department of Social Services at Wishard Memorial Hospital in Indianapolis. He is a member of the North Central Sociological Association and the American Public Health Association.

1

AN URBAN AMBULANCE SERVICE

At the intersection of two very busy city streets, an ambulance with siren wailing and red and white lights flashing slows down slightly and then proceeds through a red light while oncoming traffic in both directions comes to a temporary halt. Once across the red light at the intersection, the ambulance quickly proceeds down the crowded thoroughfare at a rate of speed that most drivers would reserve for the freeway. Curious on-lookers no doubt wonder about the destination of the ambulance, asking themselves familiar questions: "Has there been an accident? A fire? Someone sick? Injured?" If they are especially concerned, they may hope that the ambulance is not destined for their own home, office, or apartment building. If there is a patient in the ambulance and the by-standers catch a glimpse of the activity within it, they may question themselves further: "I wonder who the person is? How badly hurt? Will he or she live?" And finally exclaim to themselves, "Glad it's not me!" Such an interior monologue takes only seconds and evaporates from the mind as quickly as the ambulance disappears down the street. For many persons, if not most, this is the extent of their curiosity about ambulances and the people in them: a fleeting curiosity stimulated by occasional sightings. A smaller number will have their curiosity more actively aroused by having been transported in an ambulance, either as an emergency victim or as a friend or relative of someone requiring emergency ambulance care. For most people, however, emergency ambulance work is unfamiliar, involving activities they know little about.

The present book is about emergency ambulance work. It is an ethnography of an urban ambulance service and a description and analysis of the workaday world of the men and women who do medical work in ambulances. This study uses a sociological perspective, focusing on roles, social relationships, decision making, norms and values. It was undertaken in the hope that because of it some light might be shed on human behavior in general and human conduct in particular in medical emergencies. My hope and assumption is that many of its readers will not be professional sociologists, so the amount of sociological jargon and complex theorizing has been kept to a minimum. In order to understand better the nature of emergency ambulance work, certain sociological interpretations have been given, but my aim has been to present them in such a way that both professional and nonprofessional readers can find them interesting and enlightening.

PURPOSE AND SCOPE OF THIS STUDY

The world of emergency medical care is one of the most rapidly developing fields in present-day medicine. With respect to prehospital emergency care, the changes in this area in the past ten years have been especially astounding. As recently as the late 1960s, those who were steadily occupied in ambulance work, treating the sick and injured, had for the most part only rudimentary training in emergency medical care, and many had no training whatsoever. In the United States, the vast majority of public and private ambulance companies had virtually no requirements for hiring such workers, other than that possibly they possess strong backs and stomachs. Emergency ambulance workers were referred to in various ways as drivers, attendants, and sometimes, even more unflatteringly, as body snatchers. Primarily the basic goal of emergency ambulance work was to get to the emergency scene as quickly as possible and then to drive the victim just as quickly to the nearest hospital. Ambulances were not equipped to do much for victims beyond basic first aid; they carried little in the way of medicines or other supplies. Whatever care the victims needed to receive awaited them in the hospital emergency room and the purpose of ambulances and those who worked in them was to transport them there as rapidly as possible and keep them comfortable and quiet en route.

In the past decade that picture has changed dramatically; such television shows as "Emergency One" have made the public aware of some of these developments. Discoveries and inventions in the field of emergency medical care have had a significant impact not only on hospital energency rooms but on the prehospital setting as well. In keeping with these advances, the early 1970s saw developments at both state and federal levels to upgrade and standardize the education and training of ambulance personnel. Leading authorities in the field concluded that through education and training those who worked or wanted to work in this field could deliver some of the more sophisticated medical techniques that were then only available in hospital emergency rooms. Certification procedures were subsequently adopted by many states for emergency medical technicians (EMTs) and paramedics, requiring certain minimum qualifications in training, education, and in-service experience. Today all fifty of the United States have minimum standards that must be met in regard to the ambulances used in emergency work—their communication system, size, medical supplies and equipment—and the personnel who staff the ambulances must pass certain certification requirements. For emergency victims, all this has meant an improvement in their chance for life. Those with life-threatening illnesses or injuries have a far greater chance to survive today than they would have had a decade ago.

METHODOLOGY

The data used in this study was gathered by means of my becoming a participant observer and holding formal and informal interviews with emergency medical technicians and paramedics. Participant observation is a research method employed by some sociologists in order to discover the "everyday world" of a given group of people. Such a group might belong to a specific culture, for example, the Hopi Indians; or might share a distinctive life style, like the Amish; or behavior, juvenile street gangs; or occupation, the police. Those researchers who use this method believe it gives them a certain insight and sensitivity to the values, meanings, and definitions that the particular group studied bring to their world.

As a technique for gathering data, participant observation requires the researcher both to observe at first hand and to participate in some way in the central events of those being studied. For me, this meant that I accompanied paramedics and EMTs on their daily work routines; I rode in ambulances, transported emergency victims to hospitals, even went into private homes to help patients, and so forth. As the researcher directly observes and participates in such events and daily routines, it is expected that he or she will be objective and alert in maintaining an analytic stance. The aim of the researcher is to understand, to describe, and eventually to explain the sociological significance of the group's activities and values. The participant observer should be a good watcher and listener, never letting his or her participation become so engrossing or all-absorbing that the analytic stance is forgotten. The observer must remain objective, must be in but not of the group, if he or she is later going accurately to record, describe, and explain the world of this group of people. Of course, this is easier said than done, and one of the common pitfalls of the participant-observer method is the loss of detachment and objectivity.

This study was begun in the summer of 1978. I first became interested in doing a study of urban EMTs and paramedics because of some research I had earlier done on hospital emergency medicine. It then seemed significant to look next at emergency medical care in the prehospital setting. During the summer of 1978, I became familiar with the work of the ambulance division at County Hospital in Metro-City. Because the hospital had a reputation for developments in the field of emergency medicine, I felt it would make an ideal research site. A proposal was drawn up, and presented to County Hospital officials, and not too long a time later, permission was granted me to do the study. I was given complete freedom to conduct interviews and observe any and all phases of the work in the ambulance division. The only stipulation was that I should insure the anonymity of the hospital; thus the names of all persons, the city and the hospitals have been changed.

The main source of my data comes from the observations I made while riding in various ambulances with EMT and paramedic units, when I took the role of "known observer;" that is to say, the EMTs and paramedics were fully aware that I was a sociologist engaged in a study of their behavior and relationships. They knew I was a novice in their field, and I made no pretense of knowing anything about their work in particular or the field of medicine in general. The fact that I had conducted a field study of hospital emergency rooms a few years earlier, however, meant that I was not unfamiliar with hospital emergency rooms or my role as participant-observer, a fact that was freely shared with all in the ambulance division.

My observational routine was to ride an entire shift of duty with a district ambulance or paramedic unit, making observations about the work and whatever we encountered. Since there was a rotational system, I was able to observe many different EMTs and paramedics. As an observer, I accompanied the EMTs and paramedics on their daily rounds: emergency runs, waiting for runs in the crew room, going to eat, and getting supplies.

My observations were begun in July 1978 and continued through the fall of 1979. Approximately four hundred hours of observations were conducted. In addition to this, in-depth interviews were held with some of the more experienced paramedics. Also at various times throughout the period, informal interviews were conducted with several of the administrative officials in the ambulance division.

SETTING

The setting for this study was one of the largest cities in the Midwestern United States; in terms of population, the city that I refer to as Metro-City ranks within the twenty most-populated cities in the country. Emergency ambulance is provided by County Hospital, a 700-bed hospital, located near the central core of Metro-City, operated mainly by public funding. Within the organizational structure of County Hospital, the ambulance division is responsible for providing basic life support for all of Metro-City. There are a number of private ambulance services in the city; their work, however, is mostly limited to transporting convalescent patients; they have relatively few emergency runs. The bulk of the requests for emergency ambulance service in Metro-City is provided by the ambulance division of County Hospital.

THE AMBULANCE DIVISION

County Hospital through its ambulance division operates one of the relatively few hospital-based ambulance services in the United States. Many cities use for the transport of emergency patients a combination of private ambulance companies and fire departments for emergency response. In many metropolitan areas a fire department rescue truck staffed by EMTs will respond to the scene of an accident, fire, home injury, and the like, and initiate basic life support; the victim then if need be will be transported to a hospital emergency room by a private ambulance service. By contrast, it is the responsibility of any Metro-City emergency ambulance dispatched by County Hospital both to initiate basic and advanced life support and to transport the patient to an emergency room.

The ambulance division at County Hospital has a rather complicated structure, and in addition to its own staff—EMTs, paramedics, dispatchers, and supervisors—there are a number of administrative personnel responsible for educational and training programs, communications, public relations, and general policy decisions. The present study focuses on those persons most directly involved in providing emergency medical care.

Nationally County Hospital and its ambulance division have acquired a reputation as a leader in the development of emergency ambulance care. This is a reputation that extends back into the previous century. In the nineteenth century the hospital, using horsedrawn vehicles, had one of the first urban ambulance services in the nation. Throughout the twentieth century County Hospital has continued to operate its emergency ambulance service, and in recent decades it was the first such service to have two-way radio communication. Today its hospital-ambulance communication system is reputed to be among the most modern and sophisticated in existence. With respect to the education and training of emergency-care workers, the ambulance division provides what is considered to be among the most advanced courses of instruction for paramedics in the country.

To understand something about the world of those who are engaged in emergency ambulance work, both within and outside of their vehicles, it is necessary to look at a number of other roles, structures, and processes that comprise part of the County Hospital ambulance division. Since the EMTs and paramedics who are the subject of this study work for and through the ambulance division, a description of the operations of the division in responding to calls for emergency help must be presented.

EMERGENCY MEDICAL TECHNICIANS AND PARAMEDICS

Everyone who works in an ambulance deployed by County Hospital must be certified, according to ambulance division policy, as an emergency medical technician or paramedic. EMTs and paramedics alike receive their certification as a result of having completed certain training requirements and passing certain standard, state-administered exams. (Virtually all certified paramedics are also certified EMTs.) County Hospital considers its EMTs and paramedics qualified if they meet these state certification requirements. The division in hiring new EMTs takes into account such other individual factors as experience and willingness to work a designated shift. But at the minimum, an EMT or paramedic must be state-certified, and most EMTs employed by the ambulance division have taken and passed at least an eighty-one–hour course of instruction in basic life-support techniques, and the paramedics have taken and passed at least an eight-hundred–hour course in advanced life-support techniques plus a field internship. EMTs are accordingly trained in such basic life-support techniques as monitoring vital signs—pulse rate, heartbeat, blood pressure—administering oxygen, dressing wounds, splinting fractures, and so forth. Paramedics are trained and experienced both in administering these basic skills and in advanced life-support techniques as well, including maintaining airway (intubation), administering IV (intravenous) drugs, taking and reading electrocardiographs, and a number of other advanced life-support measures. Almost all the paramedics in the ambulance division worked for some length of time as EMTs before they advanced to paramedic status. County Hospital does not train its own EMTs (other than in its in-service training programs), and expects all EMTs hired to have already had their training elsewhere. The hospital does, however, have its own training program for paramedics, classes being composed of those applicants presently engaged in EMT work who show an aptitude for advanced training.

During the time that this study was in progress (1978–1979), there were eighty-five EMTs working actively on the streets in ambulance crews. Of that group, seventeen (20 percent) were female, and the whole group had an average length of service—defined as being employed by the ambulance division—of 2.02 years; there is a rather high rate of turnover among EMTs. The ambulance division also employed twenty-one paramedics, one of whom was female, and their average length of service was 5.09 years. In addition, there were eight experienced EMTs who worked as dispatchers for the communications unit of the ambulance division, two of whom were female having an average length of service of 5.00 years. If the average length of service seems low, it must be remembered that the EMTs and paramedics have existed for not quite fifteen years in the United States.

All EMTs and paramedics in the County Hospital ambulance division are required to work an eight-hour shift. There are three options: the first or day shift (7:00 a.m.–3:00 p.m.), the second shift (3:00 p.m.–11:00 p.m.), and the third shift (11:00 p.m.–7:00 a.m.). Normally a person will work the same shift for several years unless he or she elects to do overtime as a replacement for someone away on vacation or out with illness. Some EMTs and paramedics also work on a part-time shift while they are getting a degree, and during some semesters, they transfer to a shift more compatible with their academic schedule. Such exceptions, however, are relatively infrequent. Normally ambulance crews designate and think of each other as first-shift, second-shift, or third-shift people. To know what shift a person works is to know some of the people the person works with and something about the nature of the emergency runs that shift faces, because it is assumed that the three different shifts encounter a number of slightly yet significantly different kinds of emergency cases.

County EMTs and paramedics are expected to supply their own necessities for work. An EMT supplies his or her own uniform, flashlight, scissors, stethoscopes, street number guide, and the like. The hospital does, however, provide a heavy jacket for use during the winter months.

Whatever medical supplies or equipment are required is also provided and stored in the ambulance.

DISPATCH COMMUNICATIONS

Dispatch communications or Control as it is often called, is located at County Hospital adjacent to the administrative offices of the ambulance division. All calls for emergency ambulance assistance go through this unit. It is a large, brightly lighted, air-conditioned room in which two EMT dispatchers man a very large communications console. All the dispatchers who work in Control are EMTs with considerable street experience and possess a good knowledge of the physical map and geography of Metro-City. The communications system is extremely sophisticated and would require a rather lengthy discourse to describe. Suffice it to reiterate that two-way radio communication is maintained with every ambulance crew in the division. There also are two-way radio linkages with all seven hospital emergency rooms in Metro-City. In addition to this, district ambulances and paramedic units can "patch in" through Control and talk directly to a hospital emergency room themselves. This capability is most frequently used when a paramedic needs to consult with an emergency-room physician about some advanced life-support measure. Patients who are critically ill or injured often require a drug or some other emergency measure that a paramedic can give only with a physician's permission. Thanks to the two-way radio communication, paramedics on the scene can patch into an emergency-room physician, describe the patient's condition, and the physician can in turn give the paramedics orders or directions. Finally, Control monitors all police and fire-department communications in Metro-City in order to keep abreast of any emergencies—fires, accidents, and the like—that might require the dispatch of a medical unit.

The EMTs hired to work as dispatchers in Control are also hired for specific shifts, and their hours roughly correspond to those worked by the EMTs and paramedics who make up the ambulance crew. It is a twenty-four-hour-a-day operation.

The main duty of the dispatchers is to answer calls from people who request emergency ambulance assistance. Such calls generally come from private citizens, but they also frequently come from the police and the fire department requesting help at the scene of an accident or fire. In 1977 the ambulance division responded to more than 37,000 calls, virtually all of them coming through Control.

All communications—incoming calls, directions to ambulances and paramedic units, and so forth—are recorded on magnetic tape by two large recording consoles in dispatch communications. These tapes are kept for several days and are used for control and audit purposes. Dispatchers and EMTs are therefore careful about what they say over the two-way radio, for there is at least a three-day record of every conversation.

STAFFING THE AMBULANCES

County Hospital is mandated by state law to provide twenty-four-hour basic life-support coverage for the whole of Metro-City. This means that the ambulance division must maintain enough ambulances and trained personnel to provide emergency care to anyone who requires it within the city limits. The hospital actually exceeds its basic responsibility by additionally supplying advanced life-support care in the form of specially equipped ambulances staffed by paramedics. The paramedic ambulances are used for whatever life-threatening emergencies occur in Metro-City; they also, when requested, assist the fire departments of the several townships adjacent to Metro-City. This is not part of the mandate to County Hospital; rather it is performed in the name of community service. (As of this writing some townships are hiring their own paramedics to work as part of these local fire departments, their emergency loads seeming to warrant such specialization.)

The administration at County Hospital considers time an important factor in responding to medical emergencies, and as a result, the city is divided into seven districts which blanket the geographic limits. One ambulance is assigned to and stationed in each district, and its crew is responsible for responding to all the Control-initiated calls in that area. In addition to the seven district ambulances, which provide basic life support, three paramedic units are stationed at strategic points in Metro-City. The decision about whether an emergency situation requires a district ambulance or a paramedic unit—that is one equipped to give basic or advanced life support—is made by the dispatcher. This process will be described in more detail later. In effect, at any given moment there are seven district ambulances and three paramedic units available to respond to any medical emergency in Metro-City.

Each district ambulance is staffed by a team of two EMTs, with one acting as driver for the entire shift they share together. The three paramedic ambulances are larger vehicles, designed to transport the critically ill or injured, and they are staffed by two paramedics and one EMT, who acts as driver and general assistant at the emergency scene. EMTs and paramedics alike are assigned to a particular vehicle and district—the paramedic units are designated as I, II, and III—for a period of six weeks and then rotate to another district or paramedic unit for another six-week period.

Officials in the ambulance division maintain that the rotation system serves several functions. First, because some districts are busier than others and have heavier case loads, it helps to insure that the level of medical skill among EMTs and paramedics will remain high and consistent by having everyone work in the more demanding districts at least once or twice a year. It is also argued that since some districts have more runs than others, rotation evens out the wear and tear on the vehicles. A final rationale for rotation is that EMTs and paramedics often work overtime to fill in for colleagues in other districts who are sick or on vacation. The rotation system assures that they will have a basic knowledge of the streets in the temporarily assigned district, since they will work that area for a six-week period at least once a year. While paramedics and EMTs prefer some districts over others and know some territories better than others, rotation guarantees that before long no one will be assigned to a district that is entirely unfamiliar.

SUPERVISION

On each of the three shifts, supervision of all ambulance personnel is in the hands of a senior paramedic. (At the time of my study, all three supervisors were male, and all had had a considerable amount of experience as street paramedics before being promoted to supervisor. All three men were slightly older than most of the EMTs and paramedics, and two of them had been among the first paramedics ever trained at County Hospital.) These senior paramedics have a variety of duties. One of their principle tasks is on-site supervision, for the supervisors are expected to know something about the work performance of the ambulance personnel on their shifts. In addition to this, there is a significant administrative dimension to their work; they are responsible for scheduling work assignments and vacation leaves; taking any necessary disciplinary action; acting as liaison with higher administration; and tracking down the reason for whatever complaints may occur as the result of an ambulance run. If the Control dispatcher needs another ambulance to respond to some emergency, a supervisor's own ambulance can be pressed into service. This happens fairly often, so that the supervisors are never too far removed from their crews' activities.

Although much of their daily routine is taken up with paper work and administrative activities, supervisors like to make tours of their districts during their shift on duty. They are able to communicate with ambulance personnel by means of radio, but they usually do not like to take air time for this. If they use the radio to communicate at all, it is limited to asking for some ambulance units' location, or arranging for a meeting between them and the supervisor. Should a supervisor want to talk at length with a certain district or paramedic crew he asks them to meet him at a certain hospital, or some other agreed-upon location in the city. A supervisor can find out the whereabouts of any district ambulance or paramedic unit by simply going into Control and asking the dispatcher.

Supervisors are responsible for all runs that ambulances on their shift are sent on and are also responsible for evaluating on a yearly basis the performance of the ambulance crews. In theory, the supervisors are to see that the EMTs and paramedics uphold the highest standards of emergency life-support work. In practice, it is difficult for them to evaluate personnel on a regular basis since no supervisor can possibly respond to all the runs that might occur on his particular shift. Some runs would be almost over by the time the supervisor arrived on the scene, and while he was proceeding to it, of course, other runs would be occuring in other parts of the city. Thus the supervisor's ability to give on-site appraisals of personnel is limited and constrained by time and geography. (Also the administrative obligations of the role, such as meetings, making up work schedules, and so forth, require supervisors to spend more time at the desk and less time at the scene.) Normally during a given shift, the supervisor will respond to a limited number of runs for on-site supervision and performance appraisal and hope that over the course of a year he will be able to observe at least a few times the performance of those who report to him. As mentioned a bit earlier, since the supervisors are experienced paramedics, Control can and does dispatch them to assist at a scene if it is an especially busy time and all other units are already engaged.

Supervisors usually do some work at the scene, even when they have gone there only to observe, they rarely just stand in the background. Most onlookers would, however, not be aware that one of the paramedics was indeed a supervisor. Whatever instructions, praise, or criticism, the supervisor may have is normally saved until after the run has ended and conversation can be initiated in private, away from public view.

Relations between the supervisor and the ambulance personnel are not formal or distant. Except when he must take disciplinary action against a crew—which seldom happens—most of the interaction between the supervisor and EMTs and paramedics is informal with a great deal of joking, kidding, and light-hearted discussion. Supervisors usually issue their directives in the form of requests or suggestions. There appears to be an emphasis on egalitarian working relationships rather than on rigid bureaucratic distinctions. This can doubtless in part be attributed to the fact that all supervisors have been promoted through the ranks and still have strong friendships among the EMTs and paramedics formed while they were on the street. Also, since supervisors actively respond when needed, they must engage in the cooperative and team-oriented behavior that characterizes work at an emergency scene, and this makes it difficult for them later to maintain an authoritarian aloofness in their dealings with those under their supervision.

Since the supervisor of any shift is able to be present on only a limited number of runs, much of the work of the EMTs and paramedics is done without direct supervision. As a result, ambulance crews are accustomed to and expect to have a great deal of autonomy in their daily work routine. In this sense, much of the burden of social control of the scene falls directly on the EMTs and paramedics. They must both control and look out for each other, and this tends to put great demands upon teamwork and working together as partners since the ability of one EMT or paramedic to carry out his or her own part effectively is dependent on how his or her teammates perform theirs. No EMT or paramedic can work alone; everything must be accomplished as partners in a team. The phenomenon of teamwork and its consequences for social control are discussed later in considerable detail.

In analyzing work settings and the different occupational roles people perform, one can gain a certain insight by looking at the problematic features of the work. By problematic I mean those aspects of the work or setting that promote concern on the part of the persons involved—concern significant enough to evoke various coping or adaptive responses from those who perform the work. In the chapters that follow, the problematic features of emergency ambulance work at County Hospital is described. The various ways that EMTs and paramedics meet these problems and adapt their behavior to them is presented as well.

2

THE UNCERTAINTY IN
EMERGENCY MEDICINE

One of the central issues in the sociology of medical work is the uncertainty inherent in the practice of medicine. Beginning with the early study of a hospital research ward by René Fox and continuing through the more recent efforts of Eliot Freidson, the theme of uncertainty in medical contexts is recurrent.[1] In simplified terms, the problem of uncertainty can be described as follows. In many kinds of work that those in our society perform, the daily routines and outcomes of that work are relatively certain and predictable. Workers know pretty much what they will do, how they will do it, and what the results will be. Their work proceeds at a fairly fixed pace with formally structured methods and times in which to perform it. Decisions involved in this kind of work are routine or programmable, meaning that they are the sorts of decisions that are made daily, even hourly, and with certainty of their outcome. One example of such work that is very certain, routine, and predictable, might be public-school teaching. Schoolteachers know each morning what grade they will teach, how many students they will have, who their pupils will be (their names and social backgrounds), and what time they will appear. The teacher is so certain of his or her own students and subject matter that he or she can prepare a lesson plan in advance, and schedule events and activities for each hour and minute of the class day. In effect, there are few surprises if the teacher follows standard public-school pedagogy. There are many other kinds of work in our society that follow this pattern. Assembly-line workers in factories come to know the day's routine so well that they often become bored and alienated. They place the same kind of bolt in the same kind of frame hour after hour, day after day. Assembly-line workers know at the start of each shift exactly what they will be doing each minute and exactly what events they will confront: coffee break, lunch, dinner, etc., are fixed events falling at the same hour each day. The boredom associated with this highly certain and structured work is thought to produce in part the "blue-collar blues."

In other kinds of work that people do in general, and in medical work in particular, this certainty or expectedness of fixed events is lacking in several ways. If we look at the work of doctors, we find this to be true, and other researchers have cogently described some of these problems. Physicians face the daily uncertainty of finding out what is "wrong" with their patients, what to do for them, and what the prognosis or outcome will be. Much of the time the physician is in the dark about the past, present, and future of a patient's illness or injury. This problem is so commonplace in the practice of medicine that, according to some researchers, part of the education that physicians receive in medical school is "training in uncertainty."[2] This "training in uncertainty" refers to a set of activities and experiences in medical education that student physicians are put through or exposed to, to prepare them for the vicissitudes of the uncertainty they will face later in their practices. Coping with uncertainty is part of the socialization process physicians must go through if they are to be successful.

Doctors and nurses who staff hospital emergency departments confront on a daily basis related types of uncertainty in their work. As I reported in an earlier study, emergency-room doctors and nurses are uncertain about what kinds of emergency patients the day will bring. (Will there be a trauma, cardiac arrest, suicide attempt, drowning?)[3] Nor are they certain just when these emergencies will come in (several at once, four in one shift, none at all?). In hospital emergency rooms the medical staff are rarely able to anticipate with certainty what kinds of skills and knowledge they will be called upon to exercise at any given moment during a work shift. Emergency medicine then has all the uncertainties of medicine in general, both diagnostic and prognostic, and the additional problems associated with trying to anticipate the particular kinds of emergency cases with which it may be confronted. Unlike private medical practice, or even that occurring in a number of hospital wards, emergency victims do not make their appearance by appointment!

The emergency medical technicians at County Hospital must face many of the same sorts of uncertainty briefly described above. There are, also, still other dimensions of uncertainty peculiar to their particular kind of work. In simple terms, in ambulance work, when a shift of duty is begun, the EMTs going on duty, have little way of knowing, with any real certainty what the next eight hours will hold in store for them.

Experienced and seasoned EMTs tell the newcomers on the job to "expect anything and be prepared for everything." And indeed the less-experienced EMTs soon learn that the events of any given work day can rarely be anticipated and predicted. An EMT may find his or her morning filled with one emergency run after another, and his or her afternoon spent waiting in the crew room for a run that never comes. A paramedic eager to test his or her skills in the resuscitation of a cardiac victim may go for days without the chance of helping such a victim and then have two cardiac arrest runs in a single morning.

The working lives of EMTs are filled with uncertainty about what the immediate future will hold, and what to do for and with the emergency victims they are called to help. EMTs see themselves as helpers, but in order to be of help to others, they also must be able to help themselves and their fellow crew members in structuring the uncertainties they face. While each EMT is responsible for making his or her own decisions and carrying out his or her own duties and obligations, there are certain collective or shared strategies that EMTs learn to use in managing the uncertainties of their work; such strategies often take the form of reliance on agreed-upon, experience-generated methods. EMTs will tell you that there is no substitute for experience, and experience certainly becomes by far the most useful guide in learning what to expect and what to do. The work of the EMT and the subsequent uncertainties involved begin in the communications room. The journey into the uncertain world of emergency ambulance work must accordingly start there.

DISPATCH COMMUNICATIONS

For EMTs who come to prefer a more routine and predictable environment there is dispatch communications, generally referred to as Control. As I have already mentioned, it is located in a large, brightly lighted, airy room adjacent to the administrative offices of the ambulance division of County Hospital.

For twenty-four hours a day, the two swivel chairs in front of the communications console are occupied by two dispatchers. Experienced EMTs, these dispatchers have given up the rigors of ambulance work on the street, for the temperature-controlled, quiet, and more predictable atmosphere of Control. The dispatchers at County Hospital are hired not only because they are experienced EMTs, but also because of their geographical knowledge of Metro-City and their willingness to sit hour after hour in front of a telephone and microphone. Although some still work on the street and fill in as dispatchers on a part-time basis, most work full time and content themselves with reminiscing about their former days on the street.

Almost all emergency runs that the district ambulances and paramedic units at County Hospital respond to are initiated by and through Control. Except for those people who use the emergency telephone number by mistake (there are many who call Control to complain about their hospital bills), the majority of the calls that the dispatchers answer, are requests for emergency medical assistance. The dispatcher's job is to answer the phone, listen to the request for help, and get a short description of the nature of the problem. The dispatcher then obtains the address and telephone number of the caller. The dispatcher limits his or her conversation with the caller and does not ask for either the caller's or the victim's name. This is considered the responsibility of whatever ambulance unit is sent in response to the call. The dispatcher gets only whatever information he or she considers crucial to dispatch an ambulance to the scene. The dialogue between dispatcher and caller is serious, short, and terse. After the dispatcher is satisfied that all the information needed immediately has been obtained, he or she assures the caller that an ambulance will soon be on its way. Since the dispatcher has the caller's phone number, he or she can call later and get whatever other information may be needed by the district ambulance or paramedic unit en route. Dispatchers also call back to offer advice about first aid or other efforts that bystanders might try on the victim before the ambulance arrives. Only a small percentage of cases, however, require that the dispatcher make such a call. Whatever help the victim is to receive from the ambulance division of County Hospital is now the responsibility of the EMT or paramedic crew en route.

After a call for an ambulance has been received, the problem described, and the address and phone number obtained, the dispatcher is ready to mobilize emergency medical assistance. He or she does this by deciding which of the seven district ambulances or three paramedic units it is most appropriate to send to the scene. Since reaching the scene quickly is highly valued by all who work in the ambulance division, the dispatcher will try to send the unit nearest to the scene. Normally this means that the dispatcher will determine which district encompasses the address of the caller and will dispatch whatever unit is responsible for covering that particular district. If that district ambulance or paramedic unit is already responding to a previously dispatched run and is thus "out of service," the dispatcher must determine which of the remaining ambulances are closest to the scene. The dispatcher must use his or her knowledge of the movements of the emergency units throughout the city in order to decide which ambulance to send. If the dispatcher is unsure of the location of a particular ambulance, he or she will request the "10-20" (the location) of the crew. If the 10-20 is close enough to the scene to satisfy the dispatcher, he or she will dispatch the crew even though it takes that ambulance out of its normal district and leaves the district uncovered as it were, for another call for help might come in from that district. Sometimes an ambulance crew will assist the dispatcher and announce their 10-20 without being asked, if that crew realizes that they are nearer the scene than the normal district ambulance might be. One of the abilities that the experienced EMT or paramedic acquires in his or her work is to listen to dispatch communications while engaging in other activities, e.g., conversing with partners, transporting a patient, even talking to a sociologist! In fact, part of learning to be an EMT is gaining the ability to divide one's attention between the immediate confronting reality—i.e., talking, driving, eating—and the ever-present stream of communications sent out by Control.

When the dispatcher has decided which ambulance unit is most appropriate for the response, the dispatcher is ready to send an ambulance to the scene. EMTs and paramedics refer to this process as "giving out the run," and it is in essence the beginning of their actual work. The dispatcher notifies the various ambulance crews in the division that a run is about to be given out by pressing an alert button on the console, which gives out a distinct tone over the two-way radio in the emergency ambulance. Because EMTs and paramedics know that the tone will soon be followed by the announcement of a run, the sound usually produces a brief pause in conversation or any other activity. All communication between dispatchers and ambulance crews is always brief and to the point. Runs are given out in an almost cryptic style, taking only a few seconds to complete. Here is an example: Tone ————. "District 12 . . . 711 North Kedsey . . . Code 7." This short message is immediately followed by the dispatcher's repeating the address and the code.

One of the EMTs comprising the crew of District 12 ambulance unit must now answer the dispatcher as a signal that those in the team have understood the message and are prepared to start on the run. Usually the driver will radio to Control a repeat of the address and code at the same time that he or she is putting the ambulance into gear. The dispatcher now holds up his or her end of the dialogue by informing District 12 of the correct time. Dispatchers use military parlance when they refer to the time, e.g., 14:00 hours, 13:06, and so on, and the time they give to the ambulance crew includes the hour and the minute and marks the so-called time-out of the ambulance. The time-out designation signifies the beginning of the assignment, and from that moment on until the run is completed, both Control and the EMT crew monitor the time periods that mark the various segments of the run.

The dispatcher has now also informed the crew of their "incident number," which is the number of the run on which the crew is embarking. (Each week dispatch communications begins a new numbering of the emergency calls and thus keeps a running count of the number of runs dispatched each week.) The announcement of the beginning of the first segment of the run goes like this: after the District 12 ambulance driver has repeated the address and code, the dispatcher completes the dialogue by announcing, "District 12, your time-out is 13:27; your incident number, 473."

The EMTs in District 12 ambulance are expected to transcribe all this information—address, code, time-out, and incident number—onto a log sheet that is fastened to a clipboard, which they must keep with them at all times. The log sheet is the official record of the team's runs, and by recording this initial information on the log sheet, the run has a certain legitimate status. All this activity, from the time the call comes into Control to the time the EMT crew will respond and record it on the log sheet, takes only a very few minutes.

Dispatch communications also maintains a log sheet upon which is recorded the number of the ambulance given the run, the incident number, the code and the time-out. The initial dispatcher will now monitor the progress of the run by recording the various other time periods that mark its stages. When a district ambulance or paramedic unit arrives at the scene, the crew will inform the dispatcher, who will acknowledge this by again announcing the correct time. This is referred to as "marking on the scene," and both dispatcher and crew record the time on their log sheets, next to the time-out designation. The first temporal segment of the run is then complete. As we shall examine more closely in a later chapter, the amount of time that elapses between time-out and marking on the scene is considered highly important. This first temporal segment is referred to in the County Hospital ambulance division as "response time," or the amount of time that elapses from when the district ambulance or paramedic unit departs for the scene, and when it arrives. Response time is considered to be crucial by EMTs and paramedics, particularly if it is a life-threatening emergency. According to paramedics, a difference of two or three minutes before advanced life support is initiated can be of critical importance to the patient.

If the dispatched district ambulance or paramedic unit decides to transport the patient to a hospital emergency room, this also is announced to the dispatcher. When the ambulance arrives, the crew again reports that it has "marked on" at a particular emergency room, and the time that the dispatcher announces and that both the crew and the dispatcher record on their log sheets signifies the completion of the run.

Part of the work then of the dispatcher is to record the temporal progress of each run. The timing of each run is officially recorded and monitored, and officials in the ambulance division at County Hospital can later use these log sheets to audit and study response and transport times. For the emergency ambulance crew and the dispatcher, it means that each run exists in time as well as in space. EMTs and paramedics do their work in a world marked and defined spatially by geographic location, a territoriality of streets, routes, and shortcuts. But their world is also demarcated and defined temporally, as the ever-present dispatcher announces the times into which each run is segmented.

WAITING FOR RUNS

Although EMTs and paramedics share features in common with other emergency workers such as the police, unlike the police they do not normally seek out work. Policemen have a patrol mechanism that permits them to patrol or look for trouble when headquarters has nowhere to send them. In fact, this is part of the work that the police are expected to do to maintain law and order. It allows the policeman to fill his workdays in a structured manner, as he can so employ any time between dispatch-initiated emergency runs. Normally EMTs and paramedics do not patrol the streets looking for work. While some ambulance crews have stories about coming upon an accident or emergency-related scene and offering assistance, this is far from a daily occurrence and comprises only a small portion of their work. This means that for EMTs and paramedics a good part of their everyday routine is spent waiting for something to happen. Although they see themselves as action-oriented and define their work and "finest hours" by their responses on emergency runs, all ambulance workers must learn how to maintain a high level of patience between runs. Waiting for something to happen can create just as much strain and tension in an ambulance crew as responding to a run, and EMTs and paramedics have to find ways to cope with the tensions involved in both aspects of their work.

While waiting for a run to occur, there are several places an ambulance or paramedic crew can be. Since EMTs and paramedics are accustomed to being in their ambulance, they often stay in their vehicles. If they have "marked on station," which means that the ambulance is parked at County Hospital or some other station site in Metro-City, usually a hospital, they are very apt to sit in the ambulance, waiting for their next run to occur. That is the most popular place during the warm-weather months, as it affords them the opportunity to roll down the windows and talk with colleagues or any other passersby who might feel like having a conversation. During the winter months it is more likely that when a crew "marks on station," they will adjourn to the crew room. Each hospital in Metro-City that serves as a station for a district ambulance or paramedic unit maintains a crew room. Furnished with table, chairs, and sometimes TV and a refrigerator, these rooms are not elaborate, and their rather sparse appointments do not always encourage EMTs and paramedic units to use them unless they have to. Social life in the crew room is described in more detail later; it is sufficient to say now that recreational activities to pass the time between runs include playing cards and games of chance, talking, and watching TV. A crew may also wait for runs while en route to a destination—but not while transporting a patient—as for example, returning to station after completing a run, or going to meet a supervisor at some particular place or station.

EMTs and paramedics find ways of passing the time between runs that are of a more personal nature. Indeed some regard such waiting periods as personal time. Often one of the EMTs or paramedics has an errand in the city to attend to, and the rest of the crew is expected to honor that commitment. Usually at the beginning of a shift, the person will announce such an errand and the rest of the crew will plan accordingly. These personal errands take many forms; they include using the ambulance to go to the bank, to pay a bill, to buy a magazine or newspaper, or even to register for college courses. During these errands, the crew is expected to maintain constant communication with dispatch communications through either the two-way radio in the ambulance or the hand-held radio that one member of the crew is never without. The crew is expected to respond to any dispatch-initiated run regardless of the kind of errand being attended to. The waiting time is also often filled by crews going somewhere to eat breakfast, lunch, or dinner.

The primary responsibility of the EMTs and paramedics at County Hospital is to respond to emergency runs. EMTs and paramedics discharge this responsibility by maintaining constant communication with Control. About the most serious offense or infraction of ambulance division rules that an ambulance crew can commit is to "blow a run." This occurs when a crew or some member of the crew is out of two-way radio communication, and the dispatcher cannot locate the crew to give them the run. When this happens, the dispatcher must send another unit from outside the district. To blow a run does not occur very often, but when it does, it gives the supervisor occasion to impose a severe penalty on the ambulance crew involved. It is an event that all EMTs and paramedics dread.

As a result, EMTs and paramedics consider certain areas to be safer than others in regard to maintaining communications between runs. The inside of the ambulance is thought to be most safe, since the two-way radio is constantly in operation. Assuming that the radio is working properly, any call from dispatch will be received and responded to. Areas outside the ambulance are not as safe, unless the crew happens to be in the control room when a call comes in for their district, because the EMTs or paramedics are separated from the ambulance radio. Each ambulance crew is issued one hand-held radio, and when an EMT or paramedic leaves the ambulance, he or she must be certain either to take the radio or to be in the company of the member of the crew who is carrying it. This means that if an EMT wants to be alone for any reason during working hours, he or she must either carry the radio or remain in the ambulance. To be free from the ambulance, an EMT must be almost handcuffed to a crew-mate, via the hand-held radio, or give the other person an exact idea of where he or she can be found: "I'll be in the washroom." The requirements of constant communication with dispatch literally force crew members to be near each other at all times, and afford few opportunities for individual time or space. In this sense even "personal" errands are never private, since the other members of the crew must always go along. In the words of one paramedic, "When one person wants to do something, everybody has to do it." For an EMT to conduct personal affairs during work means sharing parts of his or her private life with the rest of the crew. This sharing of private circumstances can promote more intimate relationships among EMT and paramedic crews and further solidarity and togetherness. On the other hand, when members of a crew do not get along, or are reluctant to let each other know "their business," filling waiting time through personal activities only adds to the tensions already present in the relations among crew members.

In addition to their primary responsibilities of response, the EMTs are also expected to keep their district ambulance and paramedic units filled with necessary supplies of drugs and medical equipment. The supply room for all vehicles is located at County Hospital, making it necessary for each ambulance or paramedic unit to make at least one daily trip to County in order to replenish supplies. Usually this is accomplished at the beginning of each shift. Normally EMTs and paramedics do not object to this, as it is a way of filling in time while waiting for a run and gives those involved the chance to meet with their supervisor and to visit with the crews of the ambulance units stationed at County and whatever other crews might also be attending to business at the hospital. These are occasions for camaraderie, for catching up on news, gossip, and rumors about people and events in the ambulance division.

The EMTs and paramedic units are also responsible for seeing that their vehicles are kept in fuel and in good working condition. The ambulances are refueled at County Hospital, and there is a maintenance garage several blocks from County with mechanics on duty during the first and second shifts. Keeping their vehicles supplied, fueled, and in good mechanical condition are major concerns of EMT and paramedic crews, but normally take relatively little time to accomplish.

As a result, much of the time EMTs and paramedics are "at work"—and this is a feature they share with other kinds of emergency workers—they are not actually working, i.e., providing basic or advanced life support to the ill and/or injured. While EMTs and paramedics are action-oriented and want to respond to emergency runs, part of the uncertainty of their world is, When will a run occur or will it occur at all? The waiting time between runs can be an anxious time, regardless of the activities used to keep busy or occupied. According to a member of the administrative staff of the ambulance division, "It [the number of emergency runs] goes in cycles. Nothing for a while; then all hell breaks loose. They [the ambulance crews] get real fidgety if they haven't had a run for a while. Things get real tense because they know the bottom will drop out." While several runs usually occur during each shift for each crew, the number of runs and the kinds of emergencies vary from day to day. Part of learning to cope with the vicissitudes of EMT work then is to find ways to fill the workday. Each EMT and paramedic must learn to find his or her own pleasures and take satisfaction in a variety of shared activities, and those who can take no pleasure in the company of others while waiting for a run must soon find a new kind of work.

GOING ON A RUN

Despite the fact that EMTs and paramedics spend a considerable portion of their time waiting for something to happen, they must always be prepared to take a run. Unless a district ambulance or paramedic unit is transporting a patient or having mechanical problems with its vehicle or is "out of service" for a very limited number of other reasons, it is expected to respond to any dispatcher-initiated run. No run can be refused if the unit is considered by Control to be "in service." If a crew is eating breakfast at McDonalds and has just sat down to their meal, they must respond and either leave the food on the table or eat it hurriedly in the ambulance en route to the scene. This is a regular occurrence.

Once an EMT or paramedic crew begins a run, there are three kinds of uncertainty they must face. Uncertainty, as we have seen, is one of the problematic features of their work, and it is now centered around the following concerns: finding the emergency scene; anticipating what will confront them at the scene; and making a medical judgment about what to do for the victim.

EMTs and paramedics recognize these problem areas, and as they work together over a period of time, they develop individual and collective ways of coping with them. In this sense EMTs and paramedics are no different from the rest of humanity. Like all of us, they will not accept uncertainty for any length of time without trying to render it more predictable and manageable. A large part of our time is spent in giving structure and meaning to the uncertainties that life creates for us. EMTs and paramedics are no exception to this rule, and to understand their world we must look at the uncertainties they face and their methods for making these uncertainties more predictable and structured.

FINDING THE SCENE

Metro-City is one of America's largest and most-populated cities. Like any city of its size, there are a myriad of streets, avenues, and highways, to say nothing of thousands of addresses of homes, businesses, offices, and factories. As I have already mentioned, the ambulance division of County Hospital has helped structure the work of its EMT and paramedic units by dividing Metro-City into seven geographical districts for basic life-support coverage and three districts for advanced life-support coverage. This makes the work of the EMTs and paramedics easier since the district ambulance and paramedic units normally respond to only those emergency calls within their assigned district. During the six weeks that each crew spends in a district, there is time to learn the various landmarks, buildings, parks, and other signposts that give familiarity to that particular district and allow the ambulance teams to find their way among the network of streets and expressways to their current assignment.

One of the things that sets the experienced EMT off from the novice or rookie is his or her knowledge of the territory in the various districts. In fact each EMT measures his or her experience level not only in terms of the number and kinds of emergency patients confronted but also in terms of growing familiarity with the streets in their districts.

An EMT or paramedic who has worked in the division for a couple of years will often observe that he or she knows a particular district "like the back of my hand." For those EMT or paramedic crews who have worked together for some time, finding the scene has the least amount of uncertainty. According to one experienced paramedic: "Within forty seconds from the start of the run, we know where we are going."

Although there is no set time that all ambulance units are required to meet, each responding unit is expected to get to the emergency scene as rapidly as possible. The paramedic units have a longer response time, since there are only three units to cover the entire city. District ambulance crews have admitted to me that they strive for a six-minute response time for all runs within their particular district.

For rookie EMTs the problem of finding the emergency scene quickly is a bit more significant than for the more experienced crews. The novice driver is much more likely to depend upon his partner to offer bits and pieces of information about finding the address. He or she may also consult a pocket street guide, and senior EMTs have told me that years ago it was a standard piece of equipment for rookie EMTs to carry. On some ambulance crews, locating the street address is the principal activity of those not driving. Unless the driver knows exactly where he or she is going, the others act as navigators, since the driver is busy enough maneuvering the ambulance at high speed down city streets and highways.

Of course some sections of the city are more familiar than others because they make heavier use of ambulance services. The central business core, lower socioeconomic areas, and industrial sectors are the parts of Metro-City that ambulance crews soon learn to know pretty well, because a lot of their runs originate in them. Sometimes EMTs or paramedics are able to use personal knowledge to locate the scene, if the address is near their own home or apartment or those of friends or relatives.

Occasionally an ambulance or paramedic unit has difficulty locating an address and must request assistance from Control. This is most apt to occur if the site of the run is in an area of the city in which the ambulance units seldom travel. In that case, Control usually provides some additional location information. If, however, the dispatcher feels that the street location is more common and that the EMTs are not doing their job by properly using their pocket street guides, Control may embarrass the requesting EMT in the following way:

> *Dispatcher:* If I feel a person isn't learning the streets and asks for help too often, I'll give them help with the address by saying, "Your street guide will show you that the address can be found at. . . ." Now everybody in the county knows about it!

Even more experienced EMTs and paramedics are careful about asking Control for assistance in finding an address. They know that the dispatcher will only help those who help themselves. One paramedic who has spent several years in the ambulance division expressed his reservations about asking assistance from Control: "They [Control] get pretty put out at that it seems. You can ask them—but they act like you should know where it's at. They act like it's going to break their back to figure out where you're supposed to go!"

However, one female EMT felt that some dispatchers provide too much help on occasion. According to her, "Some dispatchers give too many directions. They assume that EMT drivers don't know anything."

Despite the give-and-take involved, the relationship between Control and the responding units generally remain peaceful. Normally when a dispatcher is sending out a rookie unit to an unusual address, he or she will provide some additional information about the location without being asked. Rookie EMTs are, however, expected to learn the districts fairly quickly. Most dispatchers do not want to use air time to give directions that they feel are unnecessary. For their part, new EMTs are anxious to learn to perform their job well and soon realize that little help can be brought to emergency victims who cannot be found quickly. For this reason and others, EMTs soon learn to find their way and avoid any unnecessary confrontations with the dispatchers in Control.

CODES

EMTs and paramedics try to anticipate what they will find at the emergency scene. This is part of their uncertainty. What will the patient be like? How badly sick or injured? What technical skills for sustaining life will be required? En route to the scene, these are the thoughts that flash through their minds as the ambulance speeds through the city. Even a vague notion of what they will confront is helpful. As one of the most experienced and respected paramedics at County put it: "It cuts down on a lot of anxiety before you get there. Also if you know it's critical—you run harder; and if it's less critical, you can take a little more time and be safer."

The ambulance division at County helps EMTs and paramedics to reduce their uncertainty by using a code system to designate the different kinds of emergency runs. These codes are very similar to those used in many urban police departments. Each code represents a category of similarly related characteristics in an emergency case. The code system used at County is structured as follows:

Code 1. Traffic Injury	Code 7. Seizure.
Code 2. Heart Attack	Code 8. Unconscious Person
Code 3. Injury in Public	Code 9. Attempted Suicide
Code 4. Injury in Home	Code 10. Burns
Code 5. OB (obstetric)	Code 11. OD (overdose)
Code 6. Sick Person	Code 12. GSW (gunshot wound)

Once a request for ambulance assistance has been telephoned into Control, the dispatcher when giving out the run will translate the description of the emergency supplied by the caller into one of the above codes. In this way the EMTs and paramedics who respond to the run are given some idea of what they can expect to find at the scene. The codes help to structure reality and reduce some of the uncertainty.

Another of the more important functions of the codes is to influence the rate of speed at which the responding ambulance unit will go en route to the scene. While every unit wants a good response time, and will always drive quickly to the emergency scene, the speed will vary, depending on the code given out by dispatch.

EMTs and paramedics feel that some codes call for a faster response than others. One of the EMTs at County summed up his feelings about the codes and response time as follows: "On certain codes, such as a Code 6 and Code 7, we'll [he and his partner] go for a good response time, but since we assume it's not a major emergency, we won't drive as fast as we can. If we know it's a Code 1 or a child injured, we'll push the throttle down harder."

The world of the EMT and paramedic is, however, not always so neatly categorized. Ambiguity and doubt are the more likely companions in emergency ambulance work, and the nature of codes is no exception. The problem for EMTs and paramedics is that not all codes are equally reliable. In fact the codes give only a partial construction of the actuality, one that can and often does prove to be wrong. According to one experienced paramedic, "You'll never know what it is until you actually see the person. You have to consider who is calling the problem in. If it is the patient's family, they might be hysterical and give inaccurate information. Or if it's an attempted suicide, the family might be covering up that aspect."

EMTs and paramedics who have been on the job for a few years consider certain codes to be more predictable of what they will find than others. Most seem to agree that the codes they can least depend upon to be accurate are Code 6 and Code 7. Unfortunately, these two codes are also among their most common runs. Normally EMTs do not expect a Code 6 or Code 7 run to be a life-threatening emergency. The bulk of such runs are for patients who have relatively minor illnesses or injuries which require transportation to a hospital but that are not considered in any way to be life-threatening. There are occasions when the patient is not what the EMTs consider to be sick or injured at all. These patients, who are referred to as "crocks," are thought to use the emergency ambulance service only to get attention or transportation to a hospital for a clinic appointment. In such cases a Code 6 or Code 7 designation overstates the seriousness of the case: the patient is neither sick nor in seizure. On the other hand, the use of Code 6 or Code 7 may well understate the serious- ness of the run, and every EMT or paramedic who has had at least a few months' street experience in Metro-City has his or her favorite horror story of responding to a Code 6, expecting to find a sick person, only to find instead a person in cardiac arrest. (In such a case, the appropriate code would have been Code 2, which would have been a paramedic run, calling for advanced life support.) In even more bizarre cases, emergency ambulance crews have been confronted by a dead person when they reached the scene of a Code 6 run.

What has gone wrong? The answer lies in the ambiguity of the work of the dispatcher. His or her duty is to make meaningful the description of the emergency victim's condition that the caller has given over the telephone. Since the dispatcher cannot see either the patient or the scene, he or she must depend on whatever information has originally been given. The experienced dispatcher, of course, realizes that whoever calls may be upset, extremely anxious, and is often clearly hysterical. The dispatcher frequently asks the caller to provide additional information. If the dispatcher has some ambivalence about the nature of what the caller has described and the caller appears to be hysterical, the dispatcher will attempt to calm the person, and get him or her to speak more coherently. Sometimes the dispatcher will ask the caller to look at the patient more closely to gain additional information.

The following incident took place one afternoon in Control: A call came in, and the dispatcher was told by a male voice that the caller's brother had been unconscious for some time. The dispatcher instructed the caller to determine if the patient was breathing by placing his hand on his brother's stomach to see if it went up and down. The dispatcher said he would hold the line while he [the caller] did this. In a minute or so, the caller was back on the line and said that his brother was breathing. The dispatcher then proceeded to give the run to a district ambulance unit and announced it as Code 8. A short time later the district ambulance crew reported to Control that the patient was dead at the scene.

The dispatcher in this instance, told me that without knowing for certain, he had thought the brother was probably dead when the man called for an ambulance, and that the caller had subsequently simply misread the breathing signs. Here the dispatcher's request for more information might have been helpful, but the caller's report was inaccurate. The dispatcher had to assume, however, that what the caller described was reliable and required a Code 8 designation.

Regardless of how questionable or unreliable the accuracy of the assignments of a code may be, all EMTs and paramedics are anxious to know the code of any run which they are dispatched to respond to, and if they fail to hear Control give it out, they will ask their partner what code it is. Most of the time, and despite the fact that they know the fallacies involved, EMTs and paramedics treat the code as a partial or preliminary medical description of actuality—a definition that will do for the time being. In this sense, a designated code is treated as if it were true. It is assumed to be so until actual events prove it otherwise. Code designation provides a validation, a legitimation, for proceeding to a scene at a certain speed. At this point it is all the EMT or paramedic units have to go on. For example, if a paramedic unit is dispatched on a Code 12 (gunshot wound), the unit will proceed to the scene as though it were indeed a gunshot wound and a life-threatening emergency. This reality will not be challenged unless upon arrival at the scene, the crew is confronted by conflicting evidence. Here is a personal example:

> I was sitting in the rear compartment of a paramedic unit as it sped down a busy street in Metro-City. I knew we had a run, but I had not heard the code. One of the paramedics was busily and intently putting together an IV setup. When I asked why, he said, "We've got a Code 12." Since the paramedics at County Hospital have standing orders to use certain measures on trauma or cardiac runs, this paramedic was making preparations. He was proceeding as if the code would indeed describe the situation that he would soon confront. As it turned out, the paramedic's efforts were not in vain as the patient had sustained a shotgun wound in the abdomen.

Codes are especially relevant for paramedic ambulance units since they respond only to certain codes. At County Hospital the paramedics are trained to give advanced life support to any patient in a life-threatening situation. They also are taught to administer certain drugs intravenously, to maintain airways (intubation), and to administer and interpret electrocardiographs, among the various other techniques of advanced life support. According to the system developed by the County Hospital ambulance division, paramedic ambulance units are used only to respond to life-threatening emergencies, the district ambulances providing basic life support. The difficulty in this system is that the dispatcher does not always know positively if an emergency victim has a life-threatening illness or injury, or not. In everyday practice, the dispatcher must make his or her judgment from the often garbled and overwrought description given by the caller. As part of Control's operating procedure, in certain cases the dispatcher will automatically send a paramedic unit. Code 2 (heart attack), Code 8 (unconscious person), Code 10 (burns), Code 11 (overdose), and Code 12 (gunshot wound) are automatically considered to be life-threatening emergencies and cause the dispatch of both a paramedic unit and a district ambulance as well. The district-ambulance crew is expected to assist the paramedic crew at the scene. If the run proves indeed to be a life-threatening situation, the paramedics will need several EMTs to assist them. Supplies and equipment need to be brought from the vehicles; questions relevant to the patient's medical background must be obtained from others at the scene; vital signs must be monitored; and assorted other assignments carried out.

The dispatcher must determine from the information the caller provides whether the patient is having a heart attack or is indeed unconscious (and not dead or merely asleep). Because dispatchers are rarely supplied with complete information, they normally must assume when someone phones to report that a person has suffered a heart attack, or is unconscious, or has taken an overdose, that the situation described is life-threatening, and it is quite appropriate for them to so assume until proved otherwise, and to designate the code as 2 or 8 and dispatch a paramedic unit. Dispatchers feel that if an error is made, it is better to err on the serious side, the agreement being that it is better to give the caller's description a life-threatening code and dispatch a paramedic unit than to give the caller's description a Code 6 (sick person) and have the district ambulance find someone in cardiac arrest. As Scheff described in his article on psychiatric diagnosis, it is felt by dispatchers that when they are in doubt, it is wiser to err on the more "serious" side.[4]

Since there are more than twice as many district ambulances as paramedic units in Metro-City, the district ambulance is usually able to arrive first at the scene and make a judgment about whether a paramedic unit is really needed. If the district ambulance EMTs feel the patient is not in a life-threatening condition, they will radio this information to Control, which will then in turn radio the paramedic unit to disregard the run and return to station. According to the statistics kept in the County Hospital ambulance division, paramedic units have runs "disregarded" about 50 percent of the time. As a result there is a heightened factor of uncertainty for the paramedics at County Hospital, because even after a run has begun, there is only about half a chance that their unit will arrive at the scene.

In addition to the code designation, the dispatchers like to be able to give out any available supplementary information to whatever district ambulance and paramedic units are en route to the scene. This is a further indication that the codes are only a preliminary definition of what is to come, and EMTs and paramedic crews alike welcome other bits and pieces of information to help them construct a more accurate picture. Occasionally a code is given out by a dispatcher as "unconfirmed." In that instance the situation represented by the code exists only as a possibility. This happens most often at the site of an accident or violent encounter when a bystander notifies the police that someone has been badly injured or perhaps shot. Prior even to their own arrival at the scene, the police may request ambulance assistance in case someone actually has a life-threatening injury. When this occurs, the dispatcher will send both a paramedic unit and a district ambulance crew to assist the police at a certain location, announcing the code as Code 12—if, for example, it were a reported gunshot wound. In such a situation the dispatcher waits for the arrival of the police on the scene to verify the seriousness of the patient's or patients' condition. The information received from the police can then be sent to the paramedic unit en route. It often happens that the police find that the victim or victims require only minor medical attention and ask the dispatcher to cancel their request for a paramedic ambulance. The following personal anecdote illustrates this process:

> One morning in communications the dispatcher gave a run to a paramedic unit and announced a Code 12. The dispatcher then advised the paramedic unit to "proceed with caution." When I asked the dispatcher why he advised the unit to use "caution," he said that the gunshot wound was not yet confirmed. "On a Code 12, they [the paramedic unit] will drive with their foot through the floorboard and there might be no need." In this case the dispatcher acted wisely as the police notified Control a few minutes later that a paramedic unit was not needed.

In the situation just described, the dispatcher gave a code consistent with the preliminary information. The dispatcher needed also a way of informing the paramedic unit that their run might be disregarded. The admonishment to "proceed with caution" was a signal to the unit that the Code 12 was unconfirmed. The paramedic unit was thereby alerted by the dispatcher to treat the run as if it were a Code 12 but to proceed at a safer pace.

REDUCING UNCERTAINTY AT THE SCENE

EMTs and paramedics face many kinds of uncertainty in their work, but nowhere is the problem of uncertainty more evident than in the situations that confront them at the emergency scene. EMTs and paramedics alike evaluate themselves in terms of what they can do for an emergency victim, and it is at the scene that the patient is finally confronted and their actual work begins. While the general public, for the most part, whether bystanders or friends and relatives of the patient, can stand there and wring their hands and hope for the best, the EMTs and paramedics are expected and want to do something. The problem then is just what to do for the patient.

Although the code designation and whatever supplementary information Control may have had to pass on has given the EMTs or paramedics a partial idea of what to expect, most of the time they only begin to exercise their medical judgment after they have seen the patient. Most simply, the work of EMTs and paramedics is, in their own words, to "stabilize" the patient and transport him or her to a hospital emergency room without causing any further injury or worsening of condition. The process in reality is far more complicated in that EMTs and paramedics must make a medical judgment about how severely ill or injured the patient actually is, and what procedures are necessary to support life before reaching the hospital emergency room. This whole process might be examined as a decision-making phenomenon and studied as one of the ways through which EMTs and paramedics attempt to make fixed medical judgments in order to reduce the omnipresent factor of uncertainty. There is, however, one variable that permeates all that the EMTs or paramedics do, and that is time. In emergency medical care in general and in the prehospital setting in particular, there is an assumption by those who work in this field that emergency patients are best off in a hospital with the definitive care that can be given there. The hospital is considered to be safer, cleaner, more sterile, better equipped and staffed, and in all other ways the best hope for an emergency victim. Thus in emergency medical work the sooner the patient gets to the hospital, the better. This means that whatever medical judgments and activities EMT or paramedic crews might make and prescribe must be carried out almost immediately. While EMTs and paramedics consider their work at the emergency scene important in stabilizing a patient's condition, they feel that they should never remain on the scene longer than necessary. Of course this stipulation is difficult to measure, and the definition of "longer than necessary" will vary from situation to situation.

EMTs and paramedics do their work in a world of uncertain time. They know through the constant reminders of Control what the time is, but they never know how much time they have. In this sense, time is indeed a commodity to be counted, measured, and even hoarded. EMTs and paramedics must reach a rapid judgment about how much time to spend on the scene, how long it will take to get a patient to an emergency room, how long a patient in cardiac arrest has been without oxygen, and the like. The temporal world of EMTs and paramedics is counted in minutes and sometimes seconds. Unlike many doctors and nurses who can make their clinical judgments about patients upon information that comes in slowly over the course of hours and days and even weeks, EMT and paramedic units are required to come to decisions about medical care on information acquired in seconds and minutes. In a world where delays of a few moments can be fatal for a patient with a life-threatening illness or injury, there is a strong sense of immediacy in whatever EMTs and paramedics do. Their judgments are made in a matter of minutes; the information they seek in order to exercise such judgment must be obtained even more swiftly. EMTs and paramedics must therefore rely to a considerable extent on whatever information is most readily available, immediate, and quickly retrievable. They cannot exercise their judgment until they have defined the situation. Their search is for situational clues, the bits and pieces of information gleaned from patient, bystanders, and setting.

SIGNS AND SYMPTOMS

A number of years ago, Eliot Freidson in analyzing the clinical practice of physicians described the process in terms of the doctor sorting out the many and varied signs and symptoms presented by patients into a relatively familiar few sets of categories with which the medical profession is familiar.[5] In effect, EMTs and paramedics do the same thing. In their work they must sort out from the raw reality of the signs and symptoms that an ill or injured emergency victim presents the categories of response that will allow them to help that individual patient. This sorting and sifting process is not, however, done in the slow, methodical, and medically sophisticated manner of the trained physician. EMTs and paramedics have neither the time nor the education. The signs and symptoms they sort through are much more stark and obvious; their categories, more simple and less refined.

In making emergency medical judgments, EMTs and paramedics evaluate signs and symptoms and information about the patient from different sources. Some sources are considered to be better than others. According to one experienced paramedic, the best sources of information are, when possible, the patients themselves:

> I get my most reliable information from the patient. Anything we get from anybody else is secondhand and bound to be screwed up.

They [relatives, bystanders, etc.] may have good intentions, but they'll louse it up every time.

Implied in this statement is the idea that EMTs and paramedics have no way of assessing the reliability of what they are told by others about the patient at the scene. In the absence of sufficient time to determine the reliability of such statements, EMTs and paramedics learn to rely on whatever information can be gleaned from the patient.

The paramedic quoted above comments further on this process:

While I'm taking a history [the medical history of the patient], I'm looking at the body and touching it. I'm trying to put physical signs together with the history.

Paramedics and EMTs consider certain vital signs and symptoms basic; they are thought to be most reliable and are usually the first sought: pulse rate, blood pressure, and heart and respiration rates. Other signs thought to be important and looked for are sweating, paleness, labored breathing, skin texture, absence or presence of pain, dilated pupils, and so on. Also considered are any obvious outer signs of injury: stab wounds, lacerations, fractures, bleeding, or other obvious body disturbances. If the patient is conscious and considered capable of answering questions, EMTs and paramedics will ask the standard medical questions: What is the history of the illness or injury? How did it come about? Are there any current medications, illnesses, and problems connected with it? Verbal answers given by the patient are quickly evaluated in light of whatever other signs the EMT or paramedic can glean. If, for example, a patient who is at home indicates that he or she is taking medication, one of the EMTs or paramedics in the crew will search the patient's house or apartment in order to record from a vial or bottle the name of the medicine and thus corroborate the patient's story.

Paramedics and EMTs look for any advantage that they may discover that will make their work easier. This is especially so because of the pressure of time on their judgments. In the world of prehospital emergency care, patients and EMTs and paramedics alike are almost always strangers to one another. Ambulance crews attend to people about whom little is known by way of personal history or background. As a result, they consider it an important find if the patient is thought to have been given previous medical help by the same EMT or paramedic crew. The following personal experience taken from my field notes illustrates this:

One evening on a paramedic run I was observing, we went to an apartment building on a Code 2 [possible heart attack]. In a small, dimly lit, and cluttered apartment, an elderly man lay on a bed complaining of chest pain. While the paramedics and EMTs examined him, one of the paramedics asked, "Didn't we pick you up before? Didn't you used to live on L Street?" The elderly man said that he had lived at that address several months ago.

Sometime later I asked the paramedic why had had asked the patient those questions. He answered, "Well, if you picked them up before, you can learn about the history and progress of the illness. It helps determine what's wrong." Another paramedic on the unit agreed with this, "If you learn you've picked them up before, the patient feels better; they'll feel more relaxed."

The preceding example points out that paramedics and EMTs want to make as much use as they can of the patient's own personal medical history. Unlike private physicians who treat the same patients on a regular basis, emergency ambulance workers have mostly fleeting encounters with strangers. Their work is made easier if they can determine a "previous patient status," and the present patient is transformed into someone about whom at least something is known. When EMTs and paramedics are able to upgrade a relationship from stranger to regular patient, it accomplishes two functions: one, it provides more data about the history of the patient, which allows them to exercise better judgment about that patient's care; two, it establishes a type of social bond that puts the patient in a more relaxed frame of mind, again making the work of EMT or paramedic somewhat easier.

RELYING ON OTHERS FOR INFORMATION

By the very nature of their employment, paramedics regularly work on patients who are either unconscious or incapable of answering questions about the causes or history of their illness or injury. Many patients are unconscious, having a seizure, disoriented, or in other ways physically traumatized. While such patients of course "give off" signs and symptoms, and the paramedics examine them for clues, more specific information about the patient that only someone else can give is needed. As one paramedic put it,

If the patient's unconscious, you get help from whoever you can. Bystanders . . . whoever.

Emergency victims are rarely found alone, and of course some emergency scenes draw huge crowds. Although, as I have already mentioned, paramedics tend to regard as somewhat suspect any information given by others at the scene, some suppliers of information are considered more reliable than others. In such instances, paramedics must rely on their own experience in assessing the actual value of the information given. While no definite hierarchy of credibility is discernible, the testimony of some people at the scene will always be more highly regarded than others. Information given by another medical authority, for example, is more likely to be trusted. If a patient's daughter is a nurse and she is at the scene, her medical history of her parent would be considered relatively reliable by paramedics. Others who are close to the patient—e.g., other family members, friends, neighbors—would also be listened to but not with the same trust as a person speaking with medical knowledge. Even friends and relatives of the patient are, however, considered more valuable sources of information than strangers or onlookers at the scene— they would probably be trusted least of all. But in the world of the paramedic very often even the least reliable sources of information must be questioned if no one else is available, and some processes of medical judgment begin with a paramedic asking, "Did anyone see what happened?"

Paramedics face daily many critically ill and injured patients, and the judgments they must make about such persons are quite literally life-and-death decisions. The paramedic units in Metro-City are called upon only in life-threatening emergencies; thus much of their work is performed on dying or what even might be considered clinically dead patients. In recent years in the United States, much has been spent on coronary heart disease and the rate at which people die of heart attacks. Many of the life-threatening runs that paramedics get in Metro-City are to victims of sudden heart attack and cardiac arrest in which the patient's heart stops beating. When a person is without heartbeat, the brain receives no oxygen, and the person is only minutes away from death. In Metro-City, County Hospital paramedics are often summoned to the scene of a cardiac-arrest victim, and when they arrive, the skill of the paramedic team is severely tested and the pressures on their medical judgments are intense.

At County Hospital, all paramedics are trained to give cardiopulmonary resuscitation (CPR) and to administer other advanced life-support measures—drugs, defibrillation, intubation—to any victim of cardiac arrest. Since this is some of the most dramatic work that paramedics perform and occasionally gives them one of their most rewarding experiences—the successful resuscitation of a cardiac-arrest victim—paramedics like to work on such cases. The omnipresent issue of uncertainty, however, looms large here; sufficient information to make a wise medical judgment is not always easily obtained.

Most of the uncertainty revolves around the decision as to when to begin resuscitation on a victim or whether to continue it if someone else on the scene has already started it. If a cardiac-arrest victim has been without heart activity for some time—usually a matter of minutes—with no medical attention, it is likely that the person's brain has been damaged beyond any reasonable hope of recovery and the person can probably be considered clinically dead. If, however, only a few minutes have elapsed, it is possible in a small percentage of cases for resuscitation to be successful and for the paramedics to achieve a "save." The term "save" is used by paramedics to denote a situation in which a patient's heartbeat returns and the patient lives long enough to be eventually discharged from the hospital. That is the problem that paramedics face with a cardiac-arrest victim: How long has the patient been without a heartbeat?

The paramedics at County Hospital have a term for this, and they refer to it as being "down." If a cardiac-arrest victim has been down for a lengthy period of time, there is no chance for a save. Much of their uncertainty stems from the fact that the patient is unable to tell them what the paramedics need to know. They must rely on others at the scene to advise them how long the patient has been down. Paramedics are reluctant to begin resuscitation on someone who has no reasonable chance of being saved. Not only this, the paramedics would need to work at the scene for what to them is a fairly long time, and thus be "out of service" and unavailable for other emergency runs, working on what is in effect a dead person. Their dilemma is further complicated by the fact that once resuscitation measures have been initiated, paramedics are mandated to continue them unless "higher authority"—usually a physician—orders them to stop. In other words, once started, paramedics must continue their efforts until they arrive at a hospital emergency room and medical authority takes over their responsibility.

The doctors and nurses who work in the seven hospital emergency rooms in Metro-City have many of the same values as the County Hospital paramedics. They also hope for the successful resuscitation of cardiac-arrest victims. On the other hand, they do not want to have clinically dead patients brought into their emergency rooms by paramedic crews. Once the emergency-room staff decides to stop resuscitation, it has a corpse on its hands and must notify the patient's family and explain the death to them.[6]

If the County paramedics are not to incur the displeasure of the emergency rooms' staffs, they must be careful to begin and continue their resuscitation efforts only on viable patients. Coming to a decision about how long a patient has been down, and whether to start resuscitation, paramedics can rely only on signs and symptoms from the patient and on whatever information others at the scene can supply. In regard to the patient, each paramedic in time learns to look for certain clues; some of them are shared in common, according to the conversation of this paramedic whom I overheard. Fixed and dilated pupils are one common sign, and of course the readings from the electrocardiograph. (The electrocardiograph [EKG] records heart activity on a tape which paramedics know how to read.) If the electrocardiograph tracing shows what is referred to as "straight line," it means that the patient has virtually no heart activity. Despite such a straight-line reading, the paramedics may begin resuscitation if they are able to determine that the patient has not been down for very long.

The more experienced paramedics feel they can make a better judgment about whether or not to begin resuscitation because their long experience gives them certain other personal clues to look for in judging down time. According to one experienced paramedic,

> Something a lot of people [paramedics] miss I think is called "lividity." When a body is in cardiac arrest and has layed in a certain position for X amount of time, the blood sinks to the lowest parts of the body. Pale top, but rosy red on the lower parts. If I see that, and they're a straight line on the EKG—I won't start.

To repeat once again, paramedics must rely on others at the scene, often close family members and friends of the victim, for information about how long the patient has been down. Experienced paramedics argue that often they cannot trust such information, since those close to the victim are often upset, hysterical, and unable accurately to assess how long before the patient's breathing stopped. In talking to a paramedic who had worked at County for a number of years, I learned that it is more often the rookie paramedic that puts too much trust in what the patient's family tells them:

> A thing that throws a lot of these new paramedics is that they'll walk in [to a patient's house] and start pumping on a guy and ask the family how long has he been down. The family will say "Five minutes—no more than five minutes." Well, my God, it took us twenty minutes to get there in the ambulance! They didn't call just because the guy was complaining of chest pains—that's when he hit the floor! They'll [paramedics] start working on him. He may be straight line on the scope, but they'll go with the family's history.

The problem of whether or not to start or continue resuscitation is further complicated by the fact that paramedic units are often called upon to assist at an emergency scene and must make their judgment in the light of a decision already made by other emergency workers. In such instances perhaps other workers have already begun CPR, and the paramedic unit must decide whether to continue these efforts or stop. This is rarely an easy decision.

One morning during a meeting of the ambulance division at which I was present, several paramedics were discussing with the medical director the problems they faced in working with volunteer firemen in the townships adjacent to Metro-City. (Often paramedic units from County were called on to assist these townships on advanced life-support cases since the townships do not have their own paramedics.) The County paramedics contended that occasionally they arrived on the scene to find that the firemen had already started CPR on someone whom the paramedics considered to be legally dead. Since they represented the "higher medical authority" at the scene, they could choose to discontinue such efforts. The paramedics complained to the director that if the victim's family was present and the fire-department volunteers had already started working on the patient, the family would feel hostile toward the paramedics if they did nothing more than announce, "It's hopeless," and leave. They felt that they were under situational pressure to continue what the firemen had begun. Otherwise, in the eyes of the patient's family, the volunteer fire department would look like heroes, and the County Hospital paramedics would seem to be a couple of coldhearted, noncaring jerks. During the meeting, the medical director advised the paramedics to use the same criteria to stop CPR as were used to start it. After the meeting, several paramedics told me that this is such a "gray area" that there are no hard and fast rules.

One more anecdote is included here to highlight further the situational uncertainties of emergency scenes and the problem of establishing the reliability of accounts given by others at the scene:

> Two paramedics told me of a run they had to a known house of prostitution in the city. A woman [the madam] let them in the door to a room where a man was lying facedown on the floor. The woman said the man had knocked on the door and asked for a glass of water. When she returned with the water, he was lying on the floor. One of the paramedics remarked to me, "We had to go to work on him because she had described a sudden onset of symptoms— even though we knew he was dead. His T-shirt was on backwards, and the pockets in his pants turned inside out. He probably had a coronary upstairs, and they brought him down to the parlor.

In this case the madam had provided the kind of information—sudden onset of symptoms—that virtually mandated that the paramedics begin resuscitation, even though her reliability as a witness was doubted as soon as the victim's odd clothing arrangement was noticed. However, once the paramedics had started resuscitation, they were obliged to continue it until they reached the hospital.

There is one category of patients which EMTs and paramedics will virtually always seek to resuscitate and that is children. In the case of a child, EMTs and paramedics rarely spend much effort trying to determine how long a patient has been down. An EMT recounted to me a recent case in which he had participated:

> We were called on a seizure code, and when we got to the house, we found a three-year-old child who had choked on some food. I could tell the moment we entered the room that he [the child] had been down for a while, and we weren't sure whether to start or not. Since it was a child, we started. I thought for a while we had a save because in the ambulance they [the paramedics] got some pulse and heartbeat, but he only lived three days.

Many researchers in medical sociology have noted the special attention and efforts the medical profession expends on children. In this respect, EMTs and paramedics are no different. One paramedic with many years of "street experience" put it this way: "We'll give a kid more leeway than an older person. They still have a relatively long life ahead of them."

When a patient is critically ill, paramedics are often confronted with the problem that others on the scene who could provide needed information are unable to do so. The relatives of the patient are upset and even at times hysterical. When this occurs, the paramedics must try both to give advanced life support to the patient and to cope with the hysterical spouse or parent. Occasionally the situation assumes almost a bizarre flavor when those whom the paramedics hoped to turn to for information to reduce uncertainty become patients themselves. The following is an account of such an incident:

> An EMT driver for a paramedic unit told me of a run they had recently. Went to the home of a man with a cardiac-arrest. He was lying on the floor of the kitchen. One of the paramedics tried to get the wife, who was very upset, to give them information about her husband's medical history. They tried to get her calmed down, but she got worse. A few minutes later, while the paramedic crew was in the kitchen working on the husband, the wife had a "stroke" and went into respiratory arrest. The paramedics radioed Control for back-up assistance, and another medic unit was dispatched. Both the wife and the husband were DOA [dead on arrival] when they got them to the emergency room.

Such events occur only rarely according to the paramedics at County Hospital, but the fact that they happen at all serves to strengthen the conviction of the experienced EMT and paramedic that relatives at the scene are not always in a suitable frame of mind to give reliable information.

Another drawback about seeking information from those close to the patient is that those who give information will also want information in return. Friends and relatives of a critically ill or injured person have their own uncertainties to cope with. They are anxious to know the prognosis for their loved one. Many of them begin their information-seeking with the paramedics or EMTs who are the first medical authorities on the scene. In this sense, there is a kind of reciprocity operating in which each side has something that the other wants and needs. Of course neither side gets completely what it wants in the exchange. EMTs and paramedics, as already stated, tend to look with suspicion upon whatever information relatives or friends of the patient are able to supply. Yet something at times can be better than nothing. Family and friends, for their part, would no doubt prefer the more sophisticated prognosis of a physician, but for the moment anything that the EMT or paramedic can provide in the way of medical information is welcome.

Most EMTs and paramedics give very little prognostic data to a victim's family or friends. In this sense the exchange of information is somewhat one-sided. This is partly due to the idea of prognostic uncertainty.[7] The paramedics themselves are usually not entirely sure about the patient's condition. They are not doctors, and their diagnostic work-up is very short and incomplete. EMTs and paramedics also do not like to spend time at the scene beyond what they consider to be medically necessary. Conversation with others is therefore kept to a minimum. As far as gaining information to reduce uncertainty is concerned, EMTs and paramedics appear to believe that it is better to receive than to give. Despite this, they will normally give a tentative appraisal, cautious and to the point.

I was observing a paramedic unit on a run to a home in a nearby township. The husband was in cardiac arrest and lying on the living-room floor. The paramedics worked on the man for some time while the wife spent most of the time on the telephone trying to locate the family doctor. The medics asked her several questions about her husband, but she appeared reluctant to come into the living room and continued to make phone calls. The paramedics decided to transport to an emergency room, and they asked the wife which hospital she would prefer. She said "Well, he has been to County for his heart, and St. Luke's for his lungs." The paramedic asked her again which one she would like them to take her husband. She asked the paramedic, "Well what's wrong? His heart or his lungs?" The paramedic answered, "I think it's his heart." The wife said, "Well take him to County, and I'll get his slippers."

In this case there was much information with which the paramedics could have supplied the woman. The patient's immediate trouble was his heart—he was in cardiac arrest: no heartbeat, pulse, or blood pressure. Also the paramedics knew that the patient had been down for so long that it was extremely unlikely that he could be resuscitated once he reached the emergency room, and therefore he had little need for his slippers. Later one of the paramedics told me that he could tell that the wife was disoriented which is why he answered her question but told her as little as possible.

There are some at the scene, of course, who have the kind of authority to ask for more information. The police often ask for and receive information about what an EMT or paramedic team saw and heard at a scene if that involves a crime or violence. Sometimes insurance investigators will have questions about an accident victim or an illness-related death. One EMT kept a personal daily log with a short description of all the runs he was involved in during his shift. When I asked him why, he said, "In case the police or insurance people need it."

SUMMARY

The world of the EMT and paramedic at County Hospital is filled with uncertainty. This uncertainty presents itself in many forms—from the dispatcher's uncertainty about what a caller states about an emergency victim to the ambulance crew's uncertainty about how best to treat a patient. The very uncertainty plays a significant part in emergency medicine, in which the problems are so diverse and the emergency occurrences so difficult to predict and plan for.

The EMTs and paramedics at County Hospital accept uncertainty as something that they must live with and adapt to. It is something that they rarely talk about or complain about in any direct way. It is, nevertheless, an underlying motif that is always there but seldom confronted directly. Part of the training that EMTs and paramedics receive no doubt prepares them to deal with the clinical uncertainty, as they are taught to make judgments about the care of emergency victims. However, most EMTs and paramedics argue that there is no substitute for actual working experience; the classroom rarely prepares them for all that they encounter. Real-life emergencies never fit the neat textbook descriptions of such illnesses and injuries. EMTs and paramedics soon discover that no two cases are exactly alike, and only experience can serve as a guide in making medical judgments when things do not exactly fit the textbook formula.

As EMTs and paramedics gain experience, they learn the many ways that uncertainty can be reduced. They learn not to take the codes at face value, to evaluate the bits and pieces of information from the dispatchers in Control, to assess the reliability of information given by those present at an emergency scene, and to weigh which physical clues that the patient presents are important. Out of the initial bewilderment of the rookie emerges the reasoned medical judgments of the experienced EMT or paramedic. There is no shortcut.

As to the uncertainty about work rhythms and the quest to determine when runs will occur, how many runs there will be and of what variety, here too experience counts for much. The seasoned EMT or paramedic acquires the ability to adapt, relax, and enjoy the company of others who play the same waiting game. For some, however, the ability to slacken tension is never fully mastered, and the uncertainty of what the day or the evening will bring manifests itself in the form of stress. This is not the only area of stress associated with emergency ambulance work, and the uncertainty often spills over into other areas of work.

3

TEAMWORK AMONG EMTs AND PARAMEDICS

One of the most interesting features about the work of human beings is that it is rarely performed alone. Men and women have always joined together in work endeavors, finding that as tasks become more complicated, successful outcomes are more likely if persons work cooperatively. Part of working together is to engage in a form of labor specialization—breaking up the more difficult and complicated tasks into smaller, more manageable units, performed by a number of persons acting in concert. Labor specialization (or the division of labor) always involves problems of cooperation, coordination, and the meshing of separate tasks in a common purpose; these seem to have been the problems faced throughout history. Yet the more sophisticated division of labor is, according to sociologists, a product of modern industrial society, and each year the specialization of work increases. The problems associated with coordinating work among various highly specialized workers appear to be very contemporary phenomena.

In no institution is the growing specialization of work and the attendant problems of working together to solve a common task more evident than in the field of medicine. In the West, the past thirty years have witnessed a virtual technological explosion in the world of medicine. The traditional role of the doctor is now fragmented into a vast array of different specialities, each one concentrating on a more limited aspect of the human anatomy or disease process. The same can be said of nursing, where the general nurse has given way to the nurse practitioner, the pediatric nurse, the public-health nurse, and so forth. Within the hospital setting each new technological development has meant the invention of a new occupational role to deliver or administer the technology to patients; hence the emergence of the inhalation therapist, the physical therapist, the laboratory technician, and of course the emergency medical technician and paramedic.

All this steadily increasing specialization has meant that within the field of health care those who would be of aid to patients must participate and coordinate their efforts with a variety of other professionals. No one nowadays works alone with exclusive jurisdiction over the patient. Writers and other experts and observers of the modern health-care scene speak of health-care teams and highlight the special problems of coordinating the diverse specialized medical roles into a common task. A very important contemporary research question in the field of medicine today is, How will all these specialists work together?

There seems also to be a need, however, for even more research on how persons in the field of health care learn to work together to accomplish their common task of helping patients. In the area of emergency medicine, the problems of coordination are especially crucial; because life-and-death medical judgments must often be made in a matter of minutes, the division of labor and the nature of cooperation must be decided well in advance. The site of an acute medical emergency is no time for a medical staff to start arguing about who is to do what for whom. The world of the EMT and paramedic makes an interesting study for those attempting to learn more about the nature of teamwork and cooperation, for it is in this emergency work as in perhaps no other that the capacity to work cooperatively is so vital to the lives and health of patients.

When the EMTs and paramedics at County Hospital begin their shift of work duty, the one thing that they can be certain of is that they will not work alone; they will have at least one partner—the EMTs, as we have seen, work in pairs in the district ambulances; two paramedics and an EMT work in groups of three in the paramedic units. Thus each person can count on at least one partner, the paramedics on two. Everything during the shift will be done together; no partner can escape the company of the other partner for more than a very few minutes. Everything must be done in tandem—working, eating, resting, waiting, and playing. While EMTs and paramedics must learn to work well together at the emergency scene in carrying out their medical tasks, they must also learn to get along during those times when they are not on a run. In many respects, this is a crucial feature of EMT and paramedic work because more time is spent away from emergency medical work than is spent on the scene. Much of the eight-hour work shift goes by waiting for runs, replenishing their vehicles with supplies and gas, getting something to eat, trying to relax. Since this is time spent in the company of one's partner or partners, satisfactory relations must be achieved in these waiting periods as well.

EMTs and paramedics recognize the importance of teamwork and the problems of finding a good partner, one that each person feels he or she can work with. Much time is spent during the periods between runs in discussing the subject of partnership—who is working with whom, how both are getting along, who is to be avoided as a partner, and who has proved to be an effective one. As we shall see later, EMTs and paramedics go to considerable lengths to retain a partner they like to work with and to avoid one they consider undesirable.

Like so many aspects of emergency ambulance work, problems are more often solved through experience than by training. After all, there is little in the training that EMTs and paramedics receive—or that anyone else receives in a health-care occupation for that matter—that prepares them to get along with or work cooperatively in a partnership with others. The subtleties of interpersonal dynamics and human relatedness are seldom if ever a major part of the curriculum of emergency training. If an EMT or paramedic is to get along and work cooperatively with others, he or she must learn to do this on the job. The older, more experienced EMTs and paramedics understand the give-and-take necessary in a stable partnership, and more important, their experience tells them not only which crew members to avoid insofar as possible as partners, but in general what kinds of traits of personality and behavior to look for in others in assessing them as partners. The rookie knows little of this, and at first must work with any and every partner assigned, and get along as best as he or she can. Only time and experience shows whom to seek out and whom to stay away from.

Before looking in more detail at the nature of teamwork and at the problems of coordination and cooperation in emergency care, it might be instructive to look more generally at the overall importance of teamwork among EMTs and paramedics in their work. To me, this overall phenomenon was demonstrated most clearly during the time-out periods, the time spent waiting for a run to occur.

As I have already mentioned, EMTs and paramedics by no means spend all their working time responding to runs. It is the nature of emergency work that while cases may occur one right after another, they do not occur with any specific regularity, and it often happens that ambulance crews have an hour or so to wait between runs. As we have seen, this waiting time is filled in various ways—eating, resting, talking with the crew's supervisor, for example—but quite often it is spent waiting in the crew room, and this is time that cannot be spent by oneself, since each member of an EMT or paramedic unit must stay in constant radio contact with dispatch communications. Of course, whichever member of the crew has been entrusted with the hand-held radio has a certain freedom of movement, but the other teammate is now literally forced to stay very close to the radio for communications, which means he or she must stay close to whoever has the radio.

The crew room affords a chance to escape from the confines of the ambulance, as well as a chance to talk to other EMTs and paramedics. It is usually a scene of some activity, especially during the first and second shifts. There is much shoptalk, small talk, joking, kidding, and various forms of horseplay. In addition a variety of games in which to join are also often available. Almost all EMTs and paramedics while in the crew room join in whatever fun, conversation, or games are in progress. With very few exceptions, everyone participates to some degree. Only an extremely few remain aloof, distant, or keep to themselves for any lengthy period of time. Those who do so are noticed and regarded with suspicion as persons worthy of distrust.

When I was a participant observer at County Hospital, it seemed as if everyone knew who the loners were, those who rarely joined in or initiated group activity. They were the individuals that others regarded as less than desirable to have as partners. When crew members talked together about whom they would avoid as a partner, the names of these loners would occur more often than not. While those who actively participated in crew-room events might also from time to time be mentioned—not in their presence, of course—as less than effective partners, the loners were almost by definition so considered. Participation in crew-room activities is not automatically an indication to EMTs and paramedics that one can get along effectively with others, but consistent aloofness is almost always considered indicative of a person's inability to be an effective partner.

The social interchange that takes place in the crew room—conversation, joking, kidding, and games—serves two basic functions. On the one hand, such activities are ways of passing time, relieving boredom, and even relieving tension. As we have seen earlier, the time spent between runs must be made to seem meaningful and worthwhile, and the activities in the crew room are in part important for this reason. We also have seen that any emergency run involves a certain level of tension, anxiety, stress, and danger. Emergency scenes are rarely pleasant and appealing, and ambulance crews often confront the most basic examples of human misery and tragedy—the sick, the dying, the mutilated. In such work, less pressurized activities are needed by EMTs and paramedics to get their minds off what they have seen, heard, and done, to escape at least temporarily from what is heartbreaking and unpleasant, and to lose oneself in something happier, less serious, and just plain fun. In this sense, the games, kidding, teasing, and conversation are little more than short escapes from unpleasant memories.

Of course some of the conversation takes the form of shoptalk, in which crewmates talk over the day's runs or piece together the facts about a case which they had worked on a day or so before. This is an attempt to establish the meaning of the event within the larger scheme of meanings associated with their work. Things happen so quickly, and EMTs and paramedics are so busy working at an emergency scene that they have little time to consider the larger ramifications of what they do. As we shall see later, emotions must be and are suppressed in favor of mechanistic technical action. But in the crew room, hours and days after the run, there is time to let the thoughts and emotions come out in the form of shoptalk, and for feelings, fears, frustrations, and hoped-for outcomes to emerge.

All these ways of passing time, relieving tension, and creating meaning through the reconstruction of events can be considered one important function of crew-room activities. The other function is a bit more subtle but no less important. It has to do with the testing and affirming of the values of teamwork, cooperation, and trust in working together. EMTs and paramedics, as we have already seen, must work and get along well together in applying the techniques of their occupation to emergency victims. In so doing, they must learn whom they can get along with and whom they can trust to be an effective partner. This can be learned on the job—under fire if you will—and it often is. But effective partners can also be determined through participation in the group-oriented activities characteristic of the crew room.

Activity in the crew room is not solitary activity. Even if a paramedic or EMT were to pick up a deck of cards and begin a game of solitaire, he or she would soon find others looking on, offering advice and counsel—and that particular paramedic or EMT had better accept the advice good-naturedly and willingly. For if he or she were to demand to be left alone to his or her own devices, those who looked on would consider themselves to have learned something about that person's willingness to accept help and get along with others.

To participate in crew-room activities is to be part of a group phenomenon. Conversations and small talk are open to all, and anyone with something to add to a topic is welcome to do so. Rarely is a conversation considered too private and personal to be shared with others, or are the conversations maintained in an aura of seriousness. Usually the humorous aspects of any situation are emphasized. Even when a serious topic is being pursued, the talk is lighthearted and informal. When rookies ask experienced crew members for advice or information, it is usually given in an off-hand, and even humorous way. When criticism is offered, this too takes the form of kidding and teasing, rather than seriously confronting another with his or her mistakes or shortcomings. These are all ways in which EMTs and paramedics test each other to see who can be counted on and trusted in a critical situation. Each person has to be able to take a certain amount of kidding, teasing, and ribbing without any show of fear, anger, or frustration. To lose one's cool in the good-natured kidding of the crew room is a sign to others that this person cannot be counted on to remain cool and detached in tension-filled emergency encounters.

Games in the crew room are also group-oriented. Card games, dice, backgammon, for example, involve participating with others. While competition is stressed and the winners take pride in their victory, the underlying motif is the willingness of each person to be engaged with others in playing games, to try one's best but to maintain composure and good nature when the game goes badly and defeat is certain. Being a good loser and an equally good and gracious winner are considered important evidences of emotional control and a respect for the feelings and efforts of others. All these value judgments are, of course, part of a more general value structure, emphasizing teamwork and the capacity to work for and with others.

BEING PARTNERS

Since no EMT or paramedic works alone, the degree to which each person likes his or her job and feels good about work performance depends to a considerable extent on one's partner. Having a good, dependable, trustworthy partner is often felt to be the crucial variable in one's own performance. A good partner, by definition, means that the work goes smoothly, competently, and in ways that are generally emotionally satisfactory. On the other hand, a bad partner contributes to an ineffective and emotionally unsatisfying work routine. As one paramedic expressed it, referring to a former partner:

I once had to work with Williams as my partner for eight months. Believe me, they were the worst eight months of my life.

What makes for a good partnership in EMT and paramedic work, and why is working well together considered so important? Although there are no fast and easy answers, clues are to be found somewhere in the nature of the work itself and the staffing arrangements peculiar to the ambulance division of County Hospital. Since the nature of emergency ambulance work is by far the more important of the two variables, it will be examined first in some detail.

Emergency medicine requires the cooperative efforts of several people making an immediate effort to help an emergency victim. Usually several things must be done together and within a matter of minutes, and therefore no single person can accomplish these tasks alone. Working with others can either go smoothly and efficiently, or it can be slightly chaotic. EMTs and paramedics want their work to go smoothly and with a minimum of problems. The patient and the emergency scene provide quite enough confusion and uncertainty, as we have already seen in Chapter 2. Paramedics and EMTs do not want a partner or teammate who adds to the confusion or uncertainty inherent in the situation. A good partner is, above all, one whose actions and demeanor are consistent, predictable, and appropriate to the occasion. EMT and paramedics whose behavior is considered inappropriate are thought to reflect badly not only on themselves but also on their team. In fact, this is an interesting dimension of their work. While each person can make certain that his or her own actions are competent and appropriate, there is no guarantee that one's partner's actions will be likewise, and whatever outcome results from inappropriate behavior is shared by the entire crew or partnership. No one is left untainted by an undesirable result.

As an experienced paramedic told me:

> You've got to be able to trust your partner. You're Siamese twins from the time you punch in until you punch out. Two acting as one. One guy can't fart without the other stinking. If one guy screws up in public, it reflects on the other one.

Another example of how one partner's actions reflect on the other occurs when a crew fails to respond to a call from the dispatcher concerning a run. Earlier this was referred to as blowing a run, and it is a circumstance feared by every ambulance crew because of the disgrace and penalties involved. While such an event is rare, it usually happens because of the negligence of one person. He or she has wandered too far from the radio, and the other partner is unable to locate the missing crewmate in time to respond to the dispatcher. The dispatcher must then send another ambulance, and both partners are held responsible and accountable for the deviance of one.

EMTs and paramedics recognize this as an occupational hazard. They have little control over it other than to work with a dependable partner if they can. Unfortunately at County Hospital, EMTs and paramedics cannot pick and choose their own partners. Normally the supervisor assigns those who are to work together without giving much thought to who wants to work with whom. Since crews work the same shift at all times and keep the same vehicle, it means that partnerships remain stable for months at a time. For the EMT or paramedic with a desirable partner, this is considered a blessing; for those with an undesirable partner, it can also be highly problematic, as demonstrated by the paramedic I quoted earlier.

EMTs and paramedics will do all they can to get along with a partner since they will most likely be working together for a long period of time. In fact, inasmuch as they work together for some months, it is possible for them to get to know about each other and overcome certain initial difficulties. In other words, what may start off as a highly incompatible relationship may evolve into a relatively harmonious one as each person learns to accommodate to and live with the other's temperament and style. This is not intended to imply that in what might be considered a good partnership, the relationship is always tranquil and rewarding, but for the most part it must at least approach that ideal. Equally important, however, is the feeling of trust that EMTs and paramedics consider crucial in a good partnership. This idea of an evolving relationship or one that builds over a period of time was described to me by one paramedic as follows:

> You know that George and I have worked together a lot lately. We're really starting to work as a team now.

For that paramedic working together and working as a team were not necessarily one and the same thing. These two partners had been working together for several weeks, but their ability to function as a team had only recently evolved. The implication here seems to be that the word "team" connotes a much more close, cooperative, and no doubt, effective relationship, than simply working together in the same ambulance.

Of course it sometimes happens that one person considers his or her partner's actions so unacceptable that the relationship is terminated before it has had a chance to mature into one that both partners find rewarding. A seasoned paramedic recounted such an incident, which had occurred earlier in his career:

> I once had a new partner come into work one day—he'd been drinking. I mean it was his first day on the job. He was a half hour late. Slept through the first run. I couldn't work with him for three months to see if I could trust him. I had to make a decision right there. I went to the supervisor.

When the EMTs and paramedics at County Hospital talked about the qualities that made an effective partner, they often used the term "trust." While no one was able to articulate completely the conditions or actions that constituted trust, their use of this phrase seems consistent with the definitions of interpersonal trust that are to be found in the research literature. In particular, Kim Giffin, in a theoretical inquiry into the dimensions of interpersonal trust has set out a set of conditions that are of help to us here. The conditions are as follows:

(1) A person (P) is relying upon another person (O).
(2) P is risking something he or she values.
(3) P is attempting to achieve a desired goal.[8]

Each of these elements seems to be part of the idea of trust for paramedics and EMTs. Their work requires them to rely on the other members of their crew to do their part in the division of labor. For example, earlier it was noted that ambulance crews must be able to trust whoever is driving to the scene. Only one person can drive at a time. The partner who is not driving must have an implicit trust that the person driving will get to the scene safely and quickly. Although the nondriver can offer help in the form of directions, it remains the responsibility of the driver to maneuver the vehicle safely and swiftly through the city streets. At the scene there are a variety of tasks that EMTs and paramedics perform on emergency patients, and the labor is divided in such a way that each member of the crew has particular assignments to carry out. Each partner must assume that the other person is indeed meeting his or her responsibilities because there is little opportunity for one person to look over his or her shoulder to make sure that things are being done correctly. The partners must rely on one another to carry out their medical duties.

Also, each paramedic and EMT is risking something he or she values. This is Giffin's second condition, and it seems appropriate to emergency ambulance work. In discussion in Chapter 1, we noted that emergency ambulance work can be highly dangerous. Paramedics and EMTs risk their lives every time they step into the ambulance to respond to a run. Scenes of crime, violence, and fires are also dangerous, and ambulance personnel run the risk of injuring themselves during such encounters. Being able to rely on one's partner or crewmate helps to reduce these risks. If an EMT or paramedic can count on his or her partner to keep calm, cool, and prepared in a dangerous situation, it reduces the risk for all. As we shall see a bit later in this chapter, one of the qualities of the undesirable partner, the worker to avoid, is the person whose actions increase the risks or dangers rather than reduce them.

And finally in Giffin's third condition, each paramedic and EMT is indeed attempting to achieve a desired goal. There are some rather clear-cut outcomes that EMTs and paramedics associate with their work. Successfully helping an emergency victim, achieving good response time, avoiding accidents, are some of the goals of emergency ambulance teams, and these goals can only be accomplished through cooperative effort. They are both individual and group achievements, because while each person may make his or her own contribution, he or she must also rely on the other member or members of the crew to do the same.

To reiterate, the trusting relationship among EMT or paramedic partners does not occur quickly or spontaneously. The relationship of trust evolves over a period of time and must be tested by experience An EMT or paramedic defines trust as that behavior revealed under fire, so to speak. Only the pressures of emergency situations can show one's partner's capacity to be relied on. Only when a series of situations involving risk, reliance, and pursuit of goals is met with mutually agreed-upon satisfactory results, will two partners feel that they trust each other. According to the EMTs and paramedics at County Hospital, trust is not a verbal agreement, but something that is demonstrated in critical emergency situations.

This is why when an EMT or paramedic is working with a trustworthy partner there is a reluctance to switch partners. A new partner can prove disadvantageous for two reasons. One, the new partner may be known already among the colleague group as someone who is not very trustworthy. And two, the new partner may be a rookie without any reputation for trust at all. In the latter case, the trustworthiness of the partnership will have to be tested out in emergency situations, and that takes time.

At County Hospital and elsewhere then, there is a certain value in keeping the same known partner, and paramedics and EMTs avoid changing partners unless they have to. The day shift (7:00 a.m.–3:00 p.m.) is the most disadvantageous because most absences occur on this shift. Ambulance personnel who need and want time-off for personal appointments and other family activities are most apt to take it then. Normally this requires a second- or third-shift person working overtime to fill in for the missing paramedic or EMT. Of course there are vacation periods, sick leaves, and other dislocations that occur on every shift. The results are the same—the forming of a new partnership that will be limited to a few days or weeks.

Nevertheless, EMTs and paramedics at County Hospital want to know who they will be working with. When an established partner is about to go on vacation, the remaining partner displays some almost anxious moments in trying to ascertain who his or her new partner will be. The conversation that follows serves as an illustration:

(In the crew room at County during the day shift, two paramedics and the EMT driver who have been partners for over a year are talking about the next day's work assignment.)

Eric: I'm not working tomorrow. Taking the day off.

Fred: I wonder who the hell they'll get to work with me?

Eric: I don't know.

Alex (an EMT): I'm not working tomorrow either.

Fred: Shit—the only person I know I'm going to be working with is me!

Partnership assignments at County Hospital are made by the supervisors in the ambulance division, and in the case of finding a replacement, the supervisors are usually only too glad to find anyone who is willing to work overtime, and little regard is given to how well the new partners will get along or work together. The paramedics and EMTs, for their part often want to know whom they are scheduled to work with before accepting an overtime assignment. Very often when a supervisor asks an EMT or paramedic if he or she would be willing to work overtime, the first question directed at the supervisor is, "Who will I work with?" If it is someone with a reputation for being a less than desirable partner, the overtime assignment may well be turned down. Often this depends on how badly the EMT or paramedic needs the money; if a person is desperate, he or she may be willing to work with almost anyone.

There is yet another way that an EMT or paramedic can avoid working with an unacceptable replacement, and that is to use the "sick call." This works only if the person in question knows in advance who his or her new partner will be. If there is at least a day's notice, the paramedic or EMT can call in sick to avoid a tour of duty with an unwanted partner. While I was at County Hospital, this tactic was mentioned to me more than once. Of course it works only for temporarily assigned partners. One's regular partner cannot be so easily avoided without causing suspicion on the part of the supervisor.

Before turning to what EMTs and paramedics define as a good partnership, it is necessary to look more closely at those traits that are seen as inhibiting a trusting relationship between partners. In simple terms, paramedics and EMTs feel that a person who is a "good" EMT or paramedic will make an effective and desirable partner. Interestingly their definitions of "good" do not concentrate all that much on a person's technical competence. While an EMT or paramedic who is technically deficient can be a difficult partner with whom to work, being technically proficient or even gifted does not guarantee that a person will make a good partner. It seems to have more to do with style, demeanor, and personality.

As in so many cases, what is good is often defined in terms of the negative or bad. In defining those characteristics that make for an ineffective EMT or paramedic, the good one is what remains as the residual. EMTs and paramedics rarely speak of the traits that they see as worthy of praise, except in the most general terms. Negative dimensions of various personnel are mentioned in the course of conversation, and one must piece together the picture of the desirable partner from the scattered traits of the person to be avoided.

One of the most prominent features of the partner no one likes to work with is excessive egoism. This is referred to in various ways as someone who is "big-headed," "out for himself," or "ego-centered." Paramedics and EMTs consider that someone who is very much self-oriented makes an ineffective worker, since they define their profession as basically collectively oriented, or one that puts the needs and interests of others ahead of their own. To the degree that an EMT or paramedic injects his or her own needs and interests into the situation ahead of the patient's, the result is an undesirable partner.

One County Hospital paramedic expressed this view in the following words:

> A lot of crews don't want to work with me because they think I'm uncooperative. Hell, they're putting their own egos ahead of their work. Some paramedics are in this line of work to satisfy their needs for action and new experience. They look forward to trying their skills even if the situation doesn't call for it. They're hot-dogs! They want to show off their skills even if it won't help the patient.

Here we see a strong collectivity orientation. Paramedic skill should not be carried out just to satisfy a need to show off or appear competent. Such skills should be used only as medically dictated.

Another County paramedic was strongly opposed to the excessive egoism he felt was characteristic of many of the partners with whom he had to work:

> The bad ones [EMTs] are in it for the thrills and glory. Here they are, brand new EMTs, and they say next week they want to be paramedics! Hell, they're "red-light freaks." If people come in who are humble, sincere—they care. You've got yourself a good med-tech. Those that are ego-centered, want to do everything their own way—as far as I'm concerned, I don't want them around. They'll get you killed. Ego-trips—that's all they're after. They usually have a big mouth too. They'll get you into trouble. If you're in people's homes, especially in certain neighborhoods, you keep your mouth shut. Don't antagonize people.

In the above quote, we see that the ego-centered partner is defined in terms of self-needs and self-interests, which at least the paramedic quoted considered an improper motivation for doing EMT and/or paramedic work. Note, also, that this type of motivation and the resulting demeanor were considered dangerous. In a situation of trust, as was described earlier, persons risk things that they value. The partner who is thought to be ego-centered cannot be trusted because he or she increases the risk since his or her actions and style can provoke aggressive behavior from others. For the paramedic quoted above, the egoistic partner represents a danger to the members of the crew.

Another paramedic revealed to me that the ego-centered EMT or paramedic can even represent a danger to the patient:

> We had a run about a year ago or so to the Westinghouse plant on the edge of the city. A guy had a cardiac arrest. It took a while, but we resuscitated him. It was cold and snowing, and I wanted to transport to the nearest hospital [Mercy] which was about four minutes away. My partner who was driving wanted to go to St. Edwards [fourteen miles away] because that was the patient's family hospital. I argued with him, but his mind was made up. He wouldn't budge. It was snowing—and the patient died en route. I feel that my partner was too damn stubborn about the whole thing.

Lack of cooperation appears to be another trait that defines the undesirable EMT or paramedic. An effective partner is one who is considered to be cooperative, amiable, and willing to get involved. In this sense, part of being cooperative is the ability to get along with one's partners. Here is the way an experienced paramedic expressed this:

> If you're at each other's throats all day, you can't do the job. If you're two people working well together, you'll be at the scene in half the time. You can't work only for the pay check or the glory. If one is like that, he destroys two people—one reflects on the other.

Cooperative behavior has also been defined as working as equals. Technically speaking, EMTs working together are status equals—no one has more formal authority to make decisions than the other. The same can be said for paramedics. Except when the supervisor is on the scene, paramedic crews work as status equals with respect to formal authority. Partners who try to assert authority over others are considered too aggressive. They are attempting to turn an equalitarian relationship into one of subordination and superordination. Others in the crew often resent this.

One of the paramedics at County was described in this way by another paramedic who had worked with him before:

> Lou is really aggressive. He's the kind of person who wants to take charge. If he thinks he can get away with it, he'll push people [EMTs and paramedics] around. What I found though was that if you stand firm he'll back down.

As I mentioned earlier in this chapter, all rookie EMTs and paramedics must "prove" themselves as good team members or partners. There is a certain status that accrues to the more experienced EMT or paramedic, and usually those who have worked at County the longest are regarded as having that one quality that all their colleagues consider most important—"street experience." By virtue of their having worked the longest, they have seen more, done more, and experienced more emergency situations. The wisdom of experience from which the senior EMT or paramedic speaks is considered as important as the books and courses that the rookie was recently exposed to in his or her training. As a result, the rookie who wants to be looked upon with favor as a desirable partner is one who willingly and even eagerly accepts the advice and counsel of his or her more experienced peers. Any newcomer to the ambulance division who thinks he or she knows all there is to know about being an EMT or paramedic will find it difficult to gain acceptance among their more experienced colleagues. In this sense, the rookie proves himself or herself a good partner by taking the role of learner. The rookie is still on trial as a partner. The training may be completed and the certification in hand, but his or her potential as a partner will be measured by their more experienced colleagues in terms of their willingness to learn while working.

In the example that follows, two experienced EMTs are discussing their third partner with whom each worked when the other had a day off.

> *Al:* She's new to the job, but she's not good at taking advice. She's always got to do things her own way.
>
> *Jerry:* She's just not going to learn what she's supposed to if she keeps that attitude. She'll face a bad situation someday, and she won't know how to respond.
>
> *Al:* Yeah, a patient will go sour, and she won't be able to handle it.

Among EMTs and paramedics the "desirable" partner is thus the one who accepts and appreciates two kinds of wisdom: the wisdom of experience on the street and the wisdom of the experienced colleague. In fact, an appreciation of one is an appreciation of the other. On the one hand, the rookie proves himself or herself worthy by becoming streetwise, by gaining wisdom through his or her own experience. And on the other hand, one demonstrates an appreciation for this value—street experience—by assuming the role of learner and seeking and accepting the advice of experienced colleagues.

If we broaden the scope here a little and shift attention from what makes for a good partner in particular, to the functions of teamwork in general, we can see some of these values in a larger perspective. In emergency ambulance work, no one carries out his or her duties alone. All things are and must be done as a team because of the nature of emergency medical care. Teammates work together and help each other in applying the techniques of their occupation to those who seek their aid. In addition to this, teammates also provide experience and knowledge to one another. In these EMT and paramedic/collegial groups, knowledge and experience are neither private nor hoarded. On the contrary, those who are respected for their wisdom and experience are those who are willing sharers and tutors. Of course, for the rookie EMT or paramedic to play the role of learner, others must be willing to play the role of mentor. Such relationships are quite common but very informal and loosely structured. Each member of an EMT partnership or paramedic team at County Hospital while I was there as observer freely sought out other more experienced crewmates for advice, information, and support. It might be argued that this is one of the most important functions of the collegial grouping: the sharing of knowledge and experience.

Sometimes the early relationships that develop between the rookie and the more experienced partner are considered crucial and of lasting importance in the career of the younger worker. Jason was a paramedic who spoke almost affectionately to me about his first partner with whom he worked in his earliest days in the County ambulance division. His partner, Lowell, was still in the division and in fact served as Jason's partner the day this conversation was held.

Jason: Did you know that I was Lowell's driver for six months? It was when I first started to work at County. I owe him everything. I wouldn't be a paramedic if it weren't for Lowell. He taught me so much. Not just about medical work. He taught me about people.

Learning from more experienced teammates takes place in a variety of settings, from the relaxed comfort of the crew room to the tension-filled atmosphere of the ambulance and emergency scene. The crew room provides many opportunities for informal conversation, and much of the good-natured banter characteristic of the crew room centers on the exchange of information. Very often this takes the form of a less-experienced EMT or paramedic describing a previous run that he or she was not sure was handled appropriately. By asking a more-experienced colleague, "What would you have done?" the opportunity for giving advice is created. Usually the advice is offered sympathetically and good-naturedly. In fact, many such learning exchanges are permeated with humor and lighthearted talk. While the experienced members of a crew like to be asked for advice, and even expect it from rookies, they are rarely willing to strike a pose as instructor or authority figure. Perhaps this is due to the emphasis among ambulance crews on equality in team and partner relationships. For the experienced crewmate to take an authoritarian stance would violate the norm of equality that the crews work so hard to maintain. Consequently, when advice is given, it is given in such a way that those who seek and those who offer remain equals, even though there is an implicit recognition of the superiority of the experienced teammate.

Advice is also sometimes given during a run, and for many relatively inexperienced EMTs and paramedics, this is thought to be extremely valuable since it combines the opportunity to receive street experience and advice from senior colleagues at one and the same time. For that matter, those things that are learned while "under the gun" are probably thought to have more lasting significance than those things learned in the crew room or classroom. The following case serves as an illustration:

During the evening shift while I was observing in one of the paramedic ambulances, we were on a run to assist the fire department of an adjacent township with a patient in cardiac arrest. I was riding in the rear compartment of the ambulance with Vic, who was an EMT taking his field practicum for his paramedic certification. While Vic was technically still an EMT, he was performing paramedic tasks under the guidance of seasoned paramedics chosen by County Hospital to act as preceptors during this practicum phase of paramedic training.

On the way to the scene Herold, the preceptor paramedic, asked Vic, "Do you want to do airway when we get there instead of me? It will be a good learning opportunity for you." Vic agreed. On the way to the scene, Herold described to Vic several points to remember when intubating a patient, such as the anatomical features of the throat, the placement of the patient's head, etc. This conversation was held competing with the noise of the siren, and the communications coming in over the dispatch radio.

At the scene, we found a middle-aged–looking man lying on his back in the small living room of his bungalow. The township fire department had begun CPR. Vic took the intubation instruments from his case and slowly inserted a tube down the patient's throat. After a few minutes he stopped, and listened to the patient's chest with his stethoscope. With a puzzled look on his face he asked Herold—who had been preparing to administer electroshock—to listen to the patient's chest. Herold administered his stethoscope and said, "I think it's OK. Did you see the vocal cords when you tubed him? If you did, it's OK."

In the above illustration, Herold provided Vic with an opportunity to practice skills recently learned in the classroom on an actual patient. Herold himself could have intubated the patient with Vic looking on as learner. The value of actual street experience is so strong among EMTs and paramedics, however, that Vic was allowed to perform the technique himself. In the ambulance on his way to the scene, Herold attempted to alleviate the anxiety of Vic by "talking through" ahead of time some of the things it was necessary to remember in establishing an airway. Note that the information was phrased as some things to remember, rather than as a recitation of what must be done, thus implicitly recognizing that Vic had already been exposed to the textbook treatment of such a case. Even in the preceptor situation described above, the aura of equality is maintained by giving advice in the form of suggestions and of things to be remembered.

On those occasions where the less experienced EMT or paramedic makes an error in judgment, advice from senior colleagues also takes the form of suggestions of alternatives rather than any overt criticism. Here is an illustration:

> While I was riding as an observer with a paramedic ambulance, we were called to the scene of a multiple-injury accident. Norm, the senior paramedic, was acting as preceptor for Charles and Gale, EMTs, who were taking their field practicum for paramedic certification. They were to practice paramedic skills on the patients at the scene under the watchful eye of Norm.
>
> After the injured patients had been stabilized and transported to Mercy Hospital, and Norm, Charles, and Gale were cleaning out the ambulance, awaiting their next run, Norm quietly asked Charles why he had started IVs in both arms of the patient he was working on. Charles replied that certain indications were present that he felt required IVs in both arms. Norm said, "Where then would you get a [blood] pressure?"
>
> Charles paused and said, "Jesus, I never thought about that."
>
> Norm went on to point out several matters related to starting IVs and ended, "It's best to start with one, and get another on if you need it, but only if it is more important than getting a pressure."

This conversation was held while both Charles and Norm were busily working together putting their ambulance back in order. Norm neither chided nor castigated Charles; he was content calmly to question, point out, and offer suggestions.

Having examined the nature of learning relationships between less-experienced and more-seasoned partners, it is also instructive to look at another subtle dimension of the ambulance team relationship. While partners can and do provide information and learning experiences for one another, they are also thought to be able on some occasions to work so well together that each partner's weaknesses are matched with the other's strengths and vice versa. This seems to be characteristic of only the most enduring partnerships, where partners have been working together for some time and consider their relationship to be one of deep mutual trust.

One experienced paramedic, William described his relationship with his earliest partner at County in this way:

> I'd come in to work and be so low I couldn't stand it. Pat would be chirping away—happy as could be. Before the day was over, he had me up.

For William, one of the features that made Pat so effective a partner was Pat's ability to infect William with his enthusiasm for the day. William might be "down," to begin the shift, feeling emotionally unprepared to work, but Pat was able to share his enthusiasm with his partner. There is a kind of complementarity of resource here in the partnerships of certain EMT and paramedic crews. On some occasions, the emotional and, as we shall see, even technical resources of one partner become shared in the partnership. What one has, both have. William, the paramedic quoted above, also pointed out that there were other occasions in their partnership when he was the one who was enthusiastic and eager to work and Pat was the one who was reluctant. When this happened, Pat became infected with William's cheerfulness.

This complementarity of resource also extends in some partnerships to technical matters, when the proficiency of one partner might offset or complement the technical shortcomings of the other. Andrew, a paramedic at County for several years on the second shift, explained this phenomenon:

> I have two regular partners on the night shift. One, Gary, is brilliant in diagnostic matters and knowing what to do with patients. Nelson is the other, and he's good in techniques like starting IVs, especially in rough situations—at night, in a wrecked car. With one partner I'm able to calm him down when he gets wound up, but the other partner calms me down.

Andrew was pointing out a very subtle relationship and function that occurs in some partnerships. Such a partnership comprises far more than working together at the scene to help a patient, according to the paramedic quoted above. To be of help to patients, an ambulance team has also to be able to help each other, and this is done in part by pooling both technical and emotional resources in such a way that the team's strengths and weaknesses offset each other. For Andrew and William, their partners were valued because of this intermeshing of resources, which allows each partner who needs to, to draw upon the emotional and even technical reserve of the other. In an occupational world of uncertainty, stress, trauma, and danger, EMTs and paramedics want to have not only a partner who can be trusted but one who has the ability to share whatever technical and emotional advantages he or she has been able to accrue. While not all partnerships are so characterized, this seems to be the ideal toward which most partnerships strive.

DIVISION OF LABOR

Before turning our attention to how EMTs and paramedics must work with others and deal with such other emergency workers as doctors, nurses, policemen, and firemen, a further brief analysis needs to be made of the formal and informal division of labor among paramedics and EMTs. Since emergency victims require several kinds of emergency techniques performed upon them, and since these techniques are often performed at once, there are rules that determine who does what and to whom. In the most general sense, all EMTs and paramedics are responsible for helping emergency victims. The nature of emergency medicine makes it difficult for there to be many formally structured, bureaucratic rules regarding the dividing of emergency tasks. In general terms, however, EMTs are responsible for those tasks related to basic life support, and paramedics are responsible for advanced life support. Within this general framework, there is a more specialized division of labor within each of the two groups.

At County Hospital the EMTs work in pairs, staffing the district ambulances. During a given tour of duty, one EMT acts as the driver and is responsible for all the functions connected with driving the ambulance to and from emergency scenes. The other partner acts as "tech" and is responsible for all decisions and judgments related to maintaining basic life support in emergency victims, the driver also acting as medical assistant to the tech. This division of labor normally prevails during an entire shift. The EMT team decides at the beginning of the shift who will drive and who will be tech. Sometimes partners will adhere to this division of labor for a week at a time and then switch roles. While EMT partners are equal in the hierarchical structure of the ambulance division, the EMT acting as tech is responsible for all medical judgments.

The paramedic teams at County Hospital also have a rather simple division of labor. Medical decisions, judgments, and emergency techniques are divided into two physioanatomical areas: one devoted to maintaining a patient's airway—matters related to the patient's capacity to breathe—and to monitoring the patient's cardiovascular system; and two, concerned with the need for and administration of IVs and drug therapy. At the beginning of each shift, paramedic partners decide among themselves, which person will handle "airway" and which will handle "drugs" for the duration of that shift.

At the scene of an emergency when there are patients with conditions that require both basic and advanced life support, the divisions of labor described above are maintained, and such victims are administered to by several people at once. While there are few formal rules for deciding who does what at a scene calling for advanced life support, EMTs are expected to act in ways that generally assist the performance of paramedics. This includes what EMTs consider the more "mundane" aspects of emergency care, such as getting information about the patient for the run sheet from the victim's relatives or friends, retrieving supplies and equipment from the ambulances, and making sure the stretchers cot is ready and at hand for patient transport. In this sense, in the treatment of a patient with a life-threatening illness or injury, one can learn who has the most decision-making authority by determining who is closest to the patient. Those in direct physical contact are responsible for making what are thought to be the more crucial judgments. As one reaches the periphery of the scene, those moving back and forth between scene and ambulance, or those doing paperwork, are responsible for the mundane activities. In the work of EMT and paramedic, one of the advantages of having the status of paramedic is that one is closer to the action in an almost literal sense. The following description serves as an illustration:

During the day shift, the paramedic unit with which I was riding was called to a multiple-injury accident on an expressway in Metro-City. There were two persons injured, one of whom was an infant.

The infant drew the attention of the paramedic crew, Allan and Chuck, after determining that the other injured victim was not badly hurt. The infant required some minutes of attention as the paramedics worked in the ambulance of a district unit that was already on the scene. The district ambulance EMTs, arriving first, had radioed for a paramedic unit because the infant was unconscious. One of the EMTs on the district unit spent several minutes retrieving equipment and supplies for the paramedics from their unit.

After Chuck and Allan decided the infant was not severely injured and was ready to be transported to a nearby emergency
room, Chuck went over to the EMT and thanked her for helping
them. The EMT responded, "Hell, all I was, was a 'go-for.'" She
appeared annoyed at herself.

Later I pointed this out to Chuck, and he remarked, "I understood how she feels. I felt the same way when I was an EMT. But
now I know I couldn't do my job without her doing hers."

While everyone has their job to do, it appears that not all personnel
are equally appreciative of the efforts of others. EMTs, for example,
want paramedics to be aware of their importance in delivering emergency
medical care. Those paramedics who most recently have moved out of the
EMT ranks and into paramedic status are thought to be the most sensitive
to the work of the EMT. The following conversation took place in the
crew room at County:

Two EMTs who were partners on a district ambulance were discussing a paramedic crew that was also stationed at County and with
whom the EMT crew often worked.

One of the EMTs remarked, "This crew is real easy to get along
with because they were recently EMTs themselves. They just grad-
uated from paramedic class a month ago. They're more grateful
for what we do. The older medics are more likely to say, 'Get out
of the way. We'll do it.' But not these guys."

In addition to the formal division of labor, there is an informal division of work that also emerges among the various emergency crews. Because each crew faces a complex variety of uncertainties, stresses, and
dangers, there are pressures to make the work easier. Each crew wants its
work to go smoothly and routinely, and therefore informal arrangements
that make the work easier are favored—informal arrangements in the sense
that they are neither written rules nor rigidly adhered to; they even have
a certain ad hoc quality to them. These work rules vary among crews,
as each team or partnership attempts to create a smooth working environment. Agreements about task assignment often extend no farther than
one's immediate partner, and may be abandoned when confronted with
a new partner who is unwilling to go along with such arrangements.

Jack and Stan, EMT partners at County provide such an example.
They had been partners for several months on a district ambulance. They
both admitted to having a strong respect for each other's ability and
enjoyed working together. One of the ways the partners facilitated their
work was to abandon the tech/driver task division, which I earlier
described. Rather than taking turns each shift or each week driving and

teching, Stan acted as permanent driver, and both Stan and Jack acted as techs. Both felt that adhering rigidly to the division of responsibility between tech and driver often complicated their work rather than making it easier. In the words of Jack:

> When we arrive at the scene, we are both technicians. We give and receive advice from each other if the case requires it. What one person overlooks about a patient, the other person might see. We think it's better for patients if we are both involved.

Stan and Jack also help each other in other mutually agreed-upon ways. Because Stan drives on every run, Jack is very conscientious about assisting with the navigational task of finding the scene and negotiating their way through traffic. At intersections, for example, Jack, who is in the right-hand front seat, watches for and alerts Stan to all traffic coming from that direction. As a result, Stan maintains, "I only have to look out the left window to see the traffic coming from that direction. This makes driving easier, and we can go faster." Also, while Stan is driving, Jack listens carefully to all radio communications that are being given out in a continuous stream. It is his responsibility to keep track of where the dispatcher is sending the various ambulances in County's fleet. This is important in case they happen to be nearer the scene than the ambulance being dispatched; they can then radio Control and request the run.

While these tasks may seem relatively inconsequential, they are actually small agreements in a division of labor that adds up to a more predictable and routine work structure for these two EMTs. In a sense, they are the basis for a partnership that both Stan and Jack consider to be effective and mutually satisfying.

Since the paramedic crews at County Hospital work in crews of three—two paramedics and one EMT driver—they have other informal rules of task assignment. My own observations found no evidence of an EMT ever performing unsupervised advanced life-support techniques. One of the most common task trade-offs among the paramedic crews concerned driving to the emergency scene. In transporting a patient to a hospital, the task of driving was always the responsibility of the EMT driver, as both paramedics would be occupied with the patient in the rear of the ambulance. Getting to the scene was also, according to the formal division of labor, the responsibility of the EMT driver. In actual practice, however, some paramedics for varying reasons sometimes wanted to drive and did so, the EMT acting as front-seat navigator. My own observations uncovered no consistent motives for this, except that some paramedics trust themselves as drivers more than others; some wanted to drive as a break in the routine; and some, no doubt, felt that they knew their way around the city so well that it would make things easier if they drove.

For example, Allan, Chuck, and Eric had been crewmates for some months, Eric acting as EMT driver. On one of the days when I was observing, all three wanted to drive the ambulance, whether on a run or on the way to a coffeehouse for lunch. All three engaged in a lot of good-natured jockeying to see who would drive. When whoever was in the driver's seat had to leave it for any reason at all, one of the others would promptly climb into the seat. Allan, one of the paramedics, twice remarked to Eric, "Sure would be nice if you let me drive."

These interchanges were conducted in good humor and with horseplay. No requests to drive or sit in front were conveyed in serious or threatening tone. While all three teammates no doubt wanted to drive, only Eric, the EMT, had a legitimate claim to do so, and he was willing on many occasions to let the others take his place. The jockeying for the position of driver had, of course, to be conducted in a nonserious way, since a display of temper or hurt feelings would be contrary to the values of maintaining one's cool and being cooperative with one's partners.

Among the paramedic crews at County whom I observed, the task of driving was left almost exclusively to the EMT assigned; on other crews certain paramedics made sure that they drove at least to the scene. No one seemed willing or even concerned to challenge this, the assumption being that if someone wanted to drive badly enough, it must fill some sort of need that person had to make the work more tolerable. As long as the driver proved trustworthy to the other crew members, no one said anything to the contrary.

SUMMARY

The paramedics and EMTs who worked for County Hospital faced many uncertainties in their work, but one thing that they could be certain of was that they would never face those uncertainties alone. Among the prerequisites for doing EMT and paramedic work is the willingness to work with others and to find ways to derive some level of satisfaction in interpersonal relationships with colleagues. All EMTs and paramedics receive a considerable amount of formal training to help them apply the techniques of emergency medical care to patients, but they get little instruction, if any, to prepare them to cope with one of the most significant aspects of their work—knowing how to get along with colleagues with whom they share the common mission of medically helping emergency victims. In the absence of such training, EMTs and paramedics must learn through practical necessity and experience gained through on-the-job experience to evaluate their coworkers and to trust their partners, if a career in ambulance work is to be engaged in at all.

4

EMTs AND PARAMEDICS AND THEIR RELATIONSHIP WITH OTHER EMERGENCY WORKERS

County Hospital paramedics and EMTs must not only learn to cooperate with one another, their own colleagues; they must also learn to work with the other groups of emergency workers in Metro-City who have their own valid claims to be of help to emergency victims. Policemen, firemen, hospital emergency-room doctors and nurses, are the three other sets of workers whom EMTs and paramedics encounter in the course of their daily round. These other groups can be neither avoided nor ignored because by virtue of their special status they too have solid and legitimate claims for carrying out procedures for and upon emergency patients. The working relationships that are maintained between EMTs and paramedic ambulance crews and these other emergency workers range from resentment and hostility to respect and close cooperation. In analyzing the working agreements that are negotiated among ambulance personnel and other emergency workers, it is helpful to start with how EMTs and paramedics define their "territory."

The paramedics and EMTs at County Hospital divide their working world into two important spatial areas: the street and the hospital emergency room. The street, as we have seen, refers to the public and sometimes private scenes of streets, expressways, factories, office buildings, and homes where EMTs and paramedics are sent to find and help emergency victims. The other part of their spatial area is the hospital emergency room where they transport their patients and their own districts where they retrieve supplies and wait for their summons to the next run. When at work in either of these areas, EMTs and paramedics alike confront others who legitimately claim jurisdiction over emergency matters in these same territories. Emergency-room doctors and nurses have control over all medical activity that takes place under their province, and the police and firemen alike claim control over all things defined as a street emergency. Because EMTs and paramedics are more recently established in their emergency medical role and because of the consequent ambiguity of their status, they must accede to the authority of these more established groups of emergency workers. In fact, about the only place over which EMTs and paramedics have considerable control is within the confines of the ambulance itself. This is shown in part by the fact that EMTs and paramedics can be and are very choosy about whom they permit to ride in their ambulances. For example, most crews limit their passengers to the emergency victim, an occasional observer, and sometimes, on rare occasions, a member of the patient's family.

Almost all occupations share in common the desire to control and shape the context in which work is performed. Paramedics and EMTs are no exception to the rule. They want to be able to exercise some control over the immediate context in which they must carry out their duties. While they have considerable autonomy with respect to many of the decisions they make, the fact remains, that in the two central areas in which they work, the jurisdiction is under the control of others. In the final analysis, the police and the fire department control the streets; the physicians and nurses, the emergency rooms. Whatever measures of control in these two areas EMTs and paramedics are able to obtain is always given, never to be taken for granted. In order to do their work, emergency ambulance crews must enlist the support and sympathy of the policemen and the physician—not vice versa. It is instructive to look at how EMTs and paramedics manage to obtain some control in these public and professional areas.

IN THE STREET

When rookie EMTs learn more about their work by getting out of the classroom into the actual world of emergency medicine, they soon discover which things will help them in their work and which will hinder them. Because their work is characterized by a great deal of uncertainty and because their limited training cannot prepare them for all that they confront, EMTs are attuned to creating advantages for themselves wherever and whenever they can. In addition, they must learn that those others who also work on the streets are themselves trying to gain advantage and maintain control over their own work space.

Among the very first of the fellow emergency workers that EMTs and paramedics encounter are the police. The police have, of course, been patrolling urban streets for many years now, and part of their exclusive jurisdiction over street activity is a result of historical custom. The greater authority that the police have, however, derives from their political and legal mandate to maintain and uphold law and order in the community. Although the police are mandated to uphold the law, much of their work can be understood in terms of their concern to maintain an orderly community; it is this concept that directs most of their daily routine and their relationship with others.

The police also respond to emergency calls, and only a few years ago were responsible for about the only medical attention an emergency victim received at the scene; in many urban areas, it was administered by them. In recent years, of course, this medical function has been taken over by trained firemen and even more by trained EMTs and paramedics.

From the police's point of view, a great many emergency medical scenes represent an affront to their concept of public order, particularly when some violation of the law is involved. In such cases, the police arrive on the scene conscious of their duty to create order and enforce law, while the EMTs and paramedics arrive to administer all things medical. For the paramedic and EMT, control of the work context becomes problematic whenever the police are present, since the police claim jurisdiction—and few would dare to dispute over the way the scene will be managed and who will do what to whom.

This is not to imply that EMTs and paramedics view the police as a threat or even a hindrance. It is rather that the presence of the police means that the members of ambulance crews must at all times take into account how their actions and aims will be perceived by the police, and that they must discover how to fit their own mission into the framework created by the police. Whether the police will be a help or a hindrance is not so much up to the former as it is to the EMTs and paramedics. The police, in a sense, are answerable to no one but themselves. Their uniformed presence at the scene gives them authority over virtually everything. In most cases, they are dispassionate toward EMT and paramedic crews, permitting them to go about their duties, insofar as those duties do not interfere with their ability to maintain public order and enforce the law.

For their part, EMT and paramedic crews cannot be neutral toward the police. They know that whatever concept they have of medical order at the emergency scene must fit into the police's concept of public and legal order, not vice versa. My own observations at County Hospital pointed to a kind of cooperative, reciprocal relationship, rather than an antagonistic one. Most police seem willingly to turn the medical care of patients over to the EMTs and paramedics, in part, because it is the one dimension of an emergency scene with which they no longer need to be concerned. EMT and paramedic teams thus provide a service to the police by removing at least one person from the scene—the emergency victim. For the police this often means that the emergency has ended and that public order has been restored.

Paramedics and EMTs recognize that in the street the police are ultimately in charge. As long as no EMT or paramedic challenges this, the police can be used in ways that make the work go more smoothly and routinely. For example, at any scene of violence or crime, or where there are elements of risk and danger, EMT and paramedic crews often find the presence of the police most welcome.

Some situations involving authority seem to be more problematic than others. Cases of personal injury in traffic accidents represent those emergencies in which the underlying tensions concerning the division of authority are prevalent. Whenever an accident interferes with the normal flow of vehicular and pedestrian traffic, the sensibilities of the police about public order seem most offended. The police try to avoid, insofar as possible, traffic jams and milling crowds. On these occasions, EMT and paramedic crews often find themselves pressured to speed up their medical routine and remove the victim as quickly as possible, so that an orderly flow of people and traffic can be restored. EMTs and paramedics feel that such pressures hinder their work and interfere with the sense of control they try to maintain. Nevertheless, authority of the police takes precedence over medical judgment. In the words of one County Hospital EMT:

> Whenever there are a lot of policemen around, you have trouble deciding who is in charge. We [EMTs] have the medical competence—but the police have seniority on the street.

A County paramedic with a number of years of experience felt that the newer and younger policemen on the force were more likely to give paramedics and EMTs considerable latitude in controlling their pace of work. This was felt to be especially true at accident sites:

> There are a few old diehards who don't want us to stay at the scene. They say, "Get those wheels rolling." But they're the old timers. They want to clear the street and get traffic going.

As I have already stated, the police are very sensitive about their authority if a crime has been committed, particularly a serious one. They expect that whatever work the EMTs and paramedics do at the scene for an emergency victim always must stay within the context and limits of the work the police must do to enforce the law.

A female EMT describes an occasion in which her crewmates incurred the wrath of the police when their work on a patient interfered with a police investigation:

> We had a run last night, where we found a woman dead of carbon-monoxide poisoning. She was lying on the floor of the garage. We thought she'd committed suicide. She was "beet red," and had burns on her wrist and hand, and we couldn't figure out where she got them. We couldn't get her mouth open to intubate her—and I ended up "bagging her" all the way to Southeast [Hospital].
>
> The husband was in the garage watching us, and didn't seem very concerned at all. He asked us when we left, "Is she going to be OK?" He didn't even come to the hospital because after we brought her in, one of the emergency-room nurses asked us where the husband was.
>
> After a while the police showed up and gave the paramedics and the doctors hell. They were really mad, because they considered it a homocide. They felt we should have called them from the scene.

While relations between emergency ambulance crews and the police remain problematic, because of the division of authority at the scene, most EMTs and paramedics try to stay in good standing with individual police. The police as a category represent an authority to contend with, as EMTs and paramedics attempt to control the context of their work. On a personal level, however, paramedics and EMTs and the police often develop close interpersonal ties and even at times form friendships. In fact, the experienced EMT and paramedics know that one way of coping with the authority demands of the police is to develop friendships among individual policemen and use this friendship to gain more authority and control over the context of their own work. One experienced paramedic expressed his relations with the police to me in this way:

> I get along good with police and firemen because I know a lot of them. Some of them I go drinking with, and others I play handball. When we get to the scene—if I know the cop—he'll let me take charge.
>
> I remember once where we had a run for a shot policeman. When we got there, I saw that I knew the cop. I said to him, "Now what have you done to yourself?" And he said, "I've been shot—don't let me die." We went to work, and I told the other police on the scene that I wasn't going to leave [transport the patient] until I had started two lines [IVs]. They let me stay, and when I told them the TV camera's lights were interfering with my work, they [the police] pushed the cameras out of the way.

Relations with the police can thus improve over time. For the above-quoted paramedic one way of controlling work at the scene was to personalize relations with the police and then use prior claims of friendship to assume authority.

Another paramedic at Central contended that the police were easiest to work with when both the police and the ambulance crew have a common stake, as well as claims of friendship. As emergency situations escalate in danger, a "consciousness of kind" emerges with all emergency workers anxious to protect others as they hope to be protected themselves:

> To me, the only time we [the police and paramedics] work together is if it's a common cause. If it's a big fire, or a sniper, or a hostage situation—we're all out there to protect each other's butt. But if it's a "personal injury accident," it turns into a rivalry. Now if they [the police] know you, they'll back you both up, if things get out of hand. If it's some guy that doesn't know you— he's just going to do his job, and that's all. If you've got a friend that's a cop, you're safe.

One of the more interesting facets to the working relationship between police and the EMT and paramedic crews occurs if a policeman himself gets hurt. When a policeman is injured he is, of course, forced into a dependent posture in his status as a patient. In this sense, he has been transformed from an object of authority to a subject to be worked on; the patient status acts rapidly as an equalizer in authority relations. On the other hand, the injured police officer's colleagues exert pressure where they can to guarantee competent and immediate medical care. According to County Hospital paramedics, the police in Metro-City are most concerned about getting their injured colleague to the hospital quickly and are reluctant to allow the ambulance unit to remain at the scene for very long in applying advanced life support. Many policemen— and firemen also—adhere to the old traditional model of emergency medicine in which little was done for a patient at the scene, in favor of a speedy delivery to the hospital.

One paramedic expressed it this way:

> When a policeman gets hurt, they get panicky. They insist that we just pick him up and run. They block off the intersection for us, and we go in signal ten [lights and siren]. They don't want us to work at the scene.

Although the police provide an escort to the hospital, their pressure in favor of rapidly transporting the victim there allows the EMT or paramedic crew little opportunity to work at the scene. In effect, the police largely control the work pace and the context; to the emergency ambulance crews involved the streets indeed belong to the police.

In addition to the police, EMTs and paramedics also share the public domain with the fire department. The firemen in Metro-City respond to emergencies in two ways. First, they respond to all fires and explosions, and if there are injured persons involved, this puts them in the company of County EMT or paramedic crews. Second, each of the fire department stations in Metro-City has a rescue truck staffed with firemen who are themselves trained EMTs. Fire department rescue trucks are dispatched to emergency scenes by the local fire department as well as by the dispatcher in Control at County Hospital. Through agreements worked out among the various agencies in Metro-City responsible for coordinating the emergency services, County Hospital dispatchers also can send a fire department rescue unit to those scenes in which the response time of a County ambulance will exceed four to six minutes.

Although firemen have complete authority at the scene of a fire, and ambulance personnel must work within their jurisdiction, their authority at strictly medical emergency scenes is more ambiguous. For example, they do not have the complete control over the streets that the police have. Yet they are a force that cannot be ignored by County ambulance teams because in Metro-City, as in many other large urban areas, the fire department has a great deal of political clout, and an emerging profession like that of EMT and paramedic needs the goodwill of all the other emergency personnel with whom it works.

Working agreements and relations between firemen and members of the County Hospital ambulance staff have never been harmonious. This can be attributed in large measure to various political squabbles between those in the upper hierarchies at the Metro-City fire department and at County Hospital. At the working level, these political disagreements manifest themselves in the form of rivalry between the fire department's rescue EMTs and the EMTs and paramedics who work for County Hospital. Much of the rivalry centered around the claims of the County EMT and paramedic crews to have reached professional status, with a corresponding contempt for the fire department EMTs who are regarded as less than professional. The County EMTs, for example, argue that the fire department's EMTs are less well trained, and are not called upon often enough to keep their technical medical skills sharp. Since the County EMTs work for a hospital, much of their professional identification is with hospital-based health-care workers, rather than with such other emergency workers on the scene as police and firemen.

No matter what the County EMTs and paramedics privately think about firemen, they cannot avoid them in their work, nor did observations on the subject, when I was an observer, reveal any overt contempt or disagreements. Since fire department rescue trucks are not equipped to transport patients, by and large their work is finished the moment the County Hospital ambulance arrives.

According to one County EMT, the relationship between the fire department workers and the County was improving:

> I feel that some of the firemen do a good job. Usually when we get there, the firemen will have already gotten the vital signs [heartbeat, blood pressure, pulse] taken and have them written down on a piece of paper for us. This really saves us some time.

For some EMTs and paramedics getting along with firemen is enhanced through strong interpersonal bonds of friendship. In this sense, working with firemen is similar to working with the police. Sometimes only personal friendship can bridge the gap that exists because of occupational rivalries and antagonisms.

While several EMTs admitted to me that the working relationship between County Hospital personnel and the fire-department EMTs was improving, one experienced paramedic confessed his dislike of working with firemen:

> If I know them personally, then I don't mind them. Some of them [firemen] I've known for years. We sort of grew up in EMS [emergency medical service] together. For the most part though, they're a bunch of political, egotistical, glory-hunting bastards. They get in the way. I'd just as soon let them take care of fires, and let me take care of medicine. I wish they felt the same way. But they want to do both.

Clearly one of the factors in Metro-City that allows closer cooperation between the EMT and paramedic crews and the police is not only the police's unqualified authority, but also the fact that the police no longer have anything to do with the medical treatment of emergency patients. To the degree that the firemen have dual responsibilities, their relationship with County EMTs and paramedics will remain, at least in the short run, somewhat strained.

AT THE HOSPITAL EMERGENCY ROOM

The other important areas for County Hospital EMTs and paramedics are the seven hospital emergency rooms in Metro-City to which they transport their emergency victims. While all seven are used, five of the hospitals during the period that I was an observer received the bulk of the emergency activity.

These hospital emergency rooms are all staffed by full-time emergency-room physicians and nurses, and at least three of them treat well over a hundred cases a day, part of this load being those patients brought in by the County Hospital paramedic and EMT teams.

The hospital domain is controlled by doctors and nurses, and emergency rooms are no different. Emergency-room nurses and physicians have their own conceptions of orderly routine, and like EMTs and all other workers, they want to control the context of their work. They too are very particular about who comes into the emergency room and for what purpose. They like to be able to structure the ebb and flow of events and activities in such a way that their conception of their goals and purposes can be realized.

Because the medical role of EMT and paramedic is so recent a development, many emergency-room nurses and doctors are not completely knowledgeable about what EMTs and paramedics actually do. But because all emergency-room staffs depend upon a flow of patients to provide them with their work, EMTs and paramedics are generally welcomed when they bring in patients. Also, inasmuch as the doctors and nurses, by virtue of their training, quite genuinely like to work on patients who have what they consider to be serious illnesses and injuries, when EMTs and paramedics transport such patients, they are very welcome indeed.

In some respects, emergency-room nurses are in the domain of the hospital emergency room what policemen are in the streets. Both occupations have a clear and precise perception of orderly routine, and one of the functions of their work is to see that everything under their control runs smoothly. While emergency-room physicians represent the ultimate authority in deciding upon the medical treatment most suitable for the patient, it is the nurses who largely control the pace of events and activities and are responsible for creating an orderly environment.

Since County EMTs and paramedics transport patients to hospital emergency rooms as part of their occupational responsibilities, they, in effect, bring patients into an environment over which they have little control. Once having reached the hospital emergency room, EMTs and paramedics must adjust their own work routines and goals to fit within the framework of medical care established by the emergency-room nurses. For example, when bringing a patient to an emergency room in Metro-City, the paramedic or EMT crew cannot immediately carry the patient into a treatment room and demand the attention of a doctor. Except for those in the most critical condition who will get the immediate attention of the whole emergency-room staff, patients must wait for the attention of a nurse, who then makes an initial assessment of the patient and then assigns a room and permits the EMTs or paramedics to proceed there with the patient.

Because for the most part the work of an EMT or paramedic crew is completed once a patient has been delivered to an emergency-room facility, most ambulance crews are anxious to have the emergency-room staff take over treatment, so that they themselves can replenish supplies, clean out their vehicle, and in other ways prepare themselves for their next run. Emergency-room nurses can help this process to go more smoothly and quickly if they give patients immediate attention and subsequent room assignment. On the other hand, an emergency-room nurse can delay the whole process by ignoring the presence of an ambulance crew, or prolonging the examination of the patient, or delaying the assignment of a room.

In the words of one experienced paramedic in referring to emergency-room nurses:

> You have to have a working rapport with them, because if you don't they can make your life miserable when you come into the emergency room with a patient. They can make you feel like a piece of dirt.

Whether emergency-room nurses intentionally create problems for paramedics and EMTs was not a subject of this study; no systematic analysis of the nursing role was undertaken. It seems to be true, however, that, for whatever reason, nurses can through their actions make the work of ambulance crews go smoothly or miserably, and most persons involved in such work are aware of the fact. In short, paramedics and EMTs need to have the goodwill and support of emergency-room nurses, and they will rarely act in ways that antagonize them.

Paramedics and EMT crews have few mechanisms to cope with the problems that arise when their relationship with emergency-room nurses causes them difficulty. One means, however, that can be used, though with caution, is the device known as the incident report. The incident report is used to record for administrative officials those occasions when rules have been violated or damage to hospital property occurs through accident or negligence, or to report any other form of staff deviance.

The following example shows an attempt by a paramedic at County Hospital to use the incident report to cope with what he considered inappropriate emergency-room behavior:

> My partner Eric and I were bringing a woman into ER. She had been injured in a domestic fight. We called in on the radio so we could let them know our ETA [estimated time of arrival] and

talk to a doctor. But we couldn't get a nurse to talk to us. When we brought the patient into the ER, the nurses acted too busy to take our report. So we filed an incident report about it—and it got to the director of nursing and some of the nurses got reprimanded. Now I guess some of the nurses feel the paramedics are out to get them.

In this case, the incident report may well have served only to alienate this paramedic crew from the emergency-room nurses at County. Although the incident report brought the matter to the attention of officials, it is highly doubtful that relationships among the nurses involved and the paramedic crew were thereby improved to any degree.

My own personal observation showed that most relationships between the nurses and ambulance crews were neither hostile nor antagonistic. In fact, there were many displays of not only cooperative exchanges but even friendly talk and sociability. At one of the Metro-City hospitals, the EMT and paramedic crew room was shared by some of the emergency-room nurses, and the nurses often ate their lunch or dinner in the crew room and joined in the conversation and games in progress.

Paramedics and EMTs at County Hospital would often argue that relations with emergency-room nurses would improve if the nurses knew more about the work of the ambulance crews and had a better understanding of their role in emergency care. To this end, EMTs and paramedics often encouraged nurses to ride with them as observers on their runs. In this sense, they not only wanted and needed cooperative working arrangements among themselves and the nurses but also wanted the nurses to show them approval. Because the role of EMT and paramedic is so comparatively recent a development in emergency medicine, emergency ambulance workers want to win the acceptance of the more established and entrenched professions—medicine and nursing. There were occasions at County Hospital when this occurred, and the following anecdote may serve as an illustration:

> In the crew room at County one evening, Williams, a paramedic, was reading a magazine waiting for a run. One of the emergency-room nurses, Sally, came in, sat down, and lit a cigarette. Sally and Williams began talking, and the subject turned to methods of intubating patients.
>
> *Sally:* The other day Evans Township brought in a young girl OD [drug overdose], and they had her intubated all wrong. I told them about it, and I asked them why they had tubed her in the first place. One of them said they were paramedics. I told them, "I would have never guessed."

The above conversation shows a form of approval for Williams and the County paramedics in general. As the emergency-room nurse, Sally, describes what she considered to be the sloppy and incompetent work of a township paramedic crew, she is implicitly acknowledging the competence of Williams and his colleagues. Note that she does not dismiss the work of all paramedics. Her phrase, "I would have never guessed," implies that she has come to expect what she considers more competent work through her association with County paramedics. After she has voiced her approval in this way, Williams inquired about her willingness to ride again on the emergency ambulance with his crew. She told him she would ride again with the team fairly soon. Here the fact that this nurse had ridden as an observer and was now showing approval further convinced Williams and others like him that their working relations with nurses will improve to the degree that nurses learn more about the daily routines and problems that EMTs and paramedics face. If a nurse is willing to "ride," she might prove more willing to be of help.

WORKING WITH DOCTORS

The work of EMTs and paramedics at County Hospital brings them into daily contact with hospital emergency-room doctors. Since the doctors represent the ultimate medical authority, paramedics and EMTs realize that they can function in their work only insofar as doctors permit them. Not too many years ago—it is still sometimes true today—the younger doctors, the interns and residents, often rode in the ambulances bringing medical aid to emergency victims. In recent years, this activity has generally been given up by doctors, who seem willing to let the EMTs and paramedics do the work.

The study of how and why this transition took place would be an important undertaking. Although doctors, by and large, have turned over much of prehospital emergency work to paramedics and EMTs, they have not relinquished their ultimate control over this phase of medical care—for example, much, if not most, of the training that EMTs and paramedics receive is given by doctors. At County Hospital all emergency medical services are under the authority of a physician. And since paramedics need "doctors and orders" to carry out many of their routines, their judgments and decisions on the scene are often shaped by the authority of an emergency-room physician. In the discussion which follows about working relations with doctors, our analysis will be confined to paramedics, because they are more vitally connected to the work of the physician.

The paramedics at County Hospital receive more than eight hundred hours of training in advanced life support. Many of the medical techniques that they learn, such as intubating patients, starting IVs, and administering drugs, would only a decade or two ago have been practices reserved exclusively for physicians. Today County Hospital paramedics perform them daily, yet the actual decision regarding the administration of such medical procedures is outside their jurisdiction. They are dependent on the orders given by an emergency-room physician. In this sense, much of the work of paramedics—at least at County Hospital—must be seen in terms of their working under the jurisdiction of emergency-room physicians.

The paramedics at County receive orders from doctors in two ways that enable them to be of help to patients. One set of orders, referred to as "standing orders," consists of those directions for medication, IVs, and other advanced techniques that have been issued in advance of any particular emergency situation. Usually these are agreements which have been worked out by the County Hospital ambulance division supervisory personnel with emergency-room physicians, in which the doctors issue a set of prearranged instructions for which they assume the ultimate responsibility. Before any paramedic begins to work at County Hospital, he or she is familiarized with all the standing orders available. The second kind of orders to which paramedics are subject are so-called field orders (my phrase) or directives about medical intervention that are given to paramedics at the emergency scene via two-way radio by a Metro-City emergency-room physician. These orders are not predetermined, and the emergency-room doctor must decide on the basis of the description of the condition of the patient supplied by the paramedics at the scene whether to issue orders at all, and if so, what kind. Normally, field orders are necessitated by those circumstances in a patient's condition not covered in the conventional standing orders.

Part of the medical judgment that County Hospital paramedics must exercise is whether the condition of a patient at the scene requires only standing orders or if field orders should be sought. County paramedics are always aware of their subordinate relationship with physicians. They are highly cognizant of the fact that as their training mandate requires they are extensions of the physician. Because much of their training is given by doctors, they learn early in their careers that the constraints of their work are set by the physician's authority: they can do no more than the profession of medicine is willing to let them. However, the very nature of their work as paramedics puts them daily in a position to be of help to patients having a vast number of emergency medical problems. Because paramedics have a strong "activist" orientation toward helping patients, and within their general frame of values wish to be of service, they for the most part want orders. They want the authority that orders give them in an emergency encounter.

In this sense, standing orders are often the preferred set of orders among County Hospital paramedics. Because they are standard, predetermined, and prearranged, they have a certain taken-for-granted quality to them. As I explained in an earlier chapter, paramedics live in a world of uncertainty. Emergency events are varied and difficult to predict and manage. As a result, paramedics like all emergency workers look for any advantage they can gain to make their work less problematic and easier to perform. Standing orders by their very nature reduce uncertainty; they can be relied on because they exist and can be used by paramedics without having to be given specific permission.

Field orders on the other hand are more difficult to manage. Their issuance cannot always be counted on. Since they depend on the willingness of an emergency-room physician to issue them, they ultimately depend on the physician's being able to cope with his or her own uncertainty. In such a situation, the physician must make a judgment about the medical treatment of a patient whom he or she has never known and cannot actually see to be carried out by a paramedic whom he or she may or may not know, and if known, may consider incapable of carrying out such orders.

Paramedics acquire much knowledge in their work that helps them to reduce uncertainty. A segment of that knowledge includes the ability to get orders from a doctor when it is felt such orders are needed. The paramedics at County Hospital soon learn that in Metro-City their ability to get field orders for an emergency victim depends upon three things: the hospital emergency room, the physician, and their own personal relationship with emergency-room physicians.

Although all three County Hospital paramedic crews transport patients to the seven hospitals in Metro-City that have active emergency rooms, the paramedics are not neutral about which emergency-room staffs they prefer to work with. At the emergency scene, the patient, if he or she is conscious, is given the choice of to which emergency room he or she wants to be transported. If the patient is unconscious, a member of the family is given the option. Once the patient or the family member has decided, the paramedic crew must seek field orders from a physician on the staff of that emergency room, if standing orders are not applicable and some further form of medication or technical effort is thought to be necessary. The paramedics must then radio in to the emergency room, describe the condition of the patient to the physician, and hope that he or she will issue the desired orders.

If the patient is unconscious and there is no family member present who has a preference, County paramedics are mandated by ambulance-division procedures to go to the nearest emergency room. However, unless the emergency scene is virtually adjacent to one of the hospitals, what constitutes the closest emergency room is very much left to the discretion of the paramedic team making the decision.

There seems to be a great deal of latitude involved. My personal observations indicated that when the decision was left to the paramedics they chose those emergency rooms where they would be most likely to get satisfactory "field orders" from a physician. More specifically, the County Hospital paramedics were apt to use one or two hospitals on a fairly regular basis because the doctors in those emergency rooms were considered more reliable about giving orders, and in addition, the paramedics felt that their daily working relationships with those physicians and nurses were satisfactory and rewarding.

While the choice of the hospital facility was felt to be important in obtaining field orders, paramedics at County were also influenced by their perceptions and evaluations of the emergency-room physicians. When paramedics face a critically ill or injured patient at an emergency scene, they not only want field orders; they also want orders that they believe are appropriate to the patient's condition. Experienced paramedics at County often felt that they knew what medication or other interventions would be most beneficial to the patient, and they hoped that the emergency-room physician's orders would not only be forthcoming but consistent with their opinion. Experience had proved to most of them that the physicians in certain hospital emergency rooms could be relied upon not only to issue orders but to give those orders that the crew itself wanted.

As I have already indicated earlier in this chapter, two emergency rooms in Metro-City received the bulk of paramedic transports of critical patients for whom field orders were sought. The paramedics considered themselves to have established a relationship of trust to physicians in these facilities, and as was the case in so many aspects of their work, once a pattern that proved helpful has been established, there is great reluctance to give it up. The paramedics at County, most of all, defined as good those things that could be counted upon as fixed and certain. In keeping with this idea, once certain physicians willingly issued field orders that were considered appropriate, the paramedics tended to continue to use the emergency rooms of those physicians.

One hospital emergency room (Mercy) was considered by most paramedics to be the preferred facility for most of their desperate cases. Paramedics argued that the physicians who staffed that particular emergency room gave them the most consistent and reliable field orders.

In fact, so strong was the working relationship between County Hospital paramedics and Mercy Hospital physicians that many paramedics felt that the Mercy Hospital emergency room was a kind of home territory. The relationship there between the paramedics and the emergency-room staff began to assume a primary quality, an emotional attachment that was felt to be deeper than mere professional cooperation. This is illustrated by the following conversation that took place one evening while I was conversing with two County paramedics:

> *Eric (to the researcher):* You know Mercy emergency room really does all it can to make us [paramedics] feel at home. They want all the trauma we'll bring them. I think they get some money for trauma research.
>
> *Victor:* Yeah, they're [the Mercy physicians] willing to let us do almost anything as a way of showing support for us.

The other hospital in Metro-City that receives a good many emergency ambulance transports is County Hospital, the employing institution. County paramedics have an ambivalent attitude toward the emergency room of the hospital that employs them. On the one hand, because they work for County Hospital—and because at least at the time of this study the paramedic crew room was adjacent to the emergency room—they feel an obligation, when it is within their discretion, to radio into County for field orders. Their employee status requires them to seek the approval and support of the doctors, nurses, and administrators of the organization for which they work. On the other hand, the County Hospital emergency room is staffed by interns and residents—in addition to some full-time staff physicians—who work in the emergency room for a limited period of time, before rotating to another clinical service.

This turnover in emergency-room physicians poses several problems for County paramedics. First, the frequent change makes it difficult to build up a reservoir of trust and confidence between doctor and paramedic. Paramedics argue that in such circumstances they are never sure what doctor will be on duty, and since the interns and residents are only in the emergency service for several weeks, they are often totally unfamiliar with the work of paramedics. Furthermore, assuming that a paramedic crew is able to establish what it considers to be a cooperative relationship with an intern or resident, that would only last as long as the particular doctor was on emergency service.

Since paramedics want to work with physicians on whom they can rely, the turnover in emergency-room doctors increases their uncertainty. In an emergency situation when a paramedic must call in for orders at County, he or she is never sure what physician will be on duty and whether orders will be given or not. Secondly, because interns and residents are, in a sense, students themselves, many County paramedics feel that some emergency-room doctors will not issue field orders because they want to treat the patient themselves. To the degree that paramedics administer drugs and perform other medical techniques, it lessens the opportunity for young physicians to "get practice" in emergency procedures and techniques. In this sense, some County paramedics feel they are in competition with interns and residents for treatment of critical patients. The following conversation highlights this dilemma:

Gordon (a senior paramedic): There are problems with the doctors here at County.

Researcher: Can you give an example?

Gordon: Well we had a run the other night—had a patient with pulmonary edema. My partner requested orders from the emergency-room resident at County. The resident wouldn't give us the order. But he did give an order for some other drugs. When we got to County, my partner asked the resident why he didn't give him the order. The resident said, "I don't give orders for patients I don't see." My partner wrote this on the patient's chart.

Of all the professional relationships with which paramedics must deal, it is the relationship with the emergency-room physician that is most crucial. As an emerging profession, the extent to which paramedics can control the content of their work and expand their technical base in the field of emergency medical care depends in large measure on whether the profession of medicine permits this to occur. Because physicians represent the final medical authority and responsibility, the work of the paramedic exists at their sufferance. County paramedics are well aware that they need the support and backing of the medical profession, and go to considerable lengths to see that their actions do not infringe or threaten the authority of the physicians in Metro-City.

Despite this, my own interviews and observations indicated a certain ambivalence among paramedics concerning the physician's authority. While they realized that this authority cannot be challenged, they desired more recognition from physicians that the emergency medical work they perform at the scene is valuable, and that their own knowledge of advance life-support medicine is often superior to that of many physicians. In short, while County paramedics have no desire to replace emergency-room physicians, they would like more latitude in making emergency medical decisions. In asking for field orders, for instance, paramedics often feel that their assessments and judgments concerning the patient should be given more weight by emergency-room physicians. This feeling in part derives from the perspective of the paramedic that there is an important distinction between hospital medicine and street medicine.

Although paramedics acknowledge that emergency-room physicians have superior competence within their own hospital region, this is not a competence that can easily be transferred to street work. Paramedics consider that they themselves have a superior knowledge about street conditions and situations, which makes the practice of medical emergency care more inherently different from that practiced elsewhere. Part of the ambivalency then that paramedics hold is that physicians have so little experience and understanding of the vicissitudes of street medicine and that this prevents them from utilizing paramedic skills.

In some respects, the problem of trying to establish a solid basis for cooperative work between paramedics and emergency-room physicians is similar to their dilemma with nurses. Paramedics feel that greater cooperation is possible if physicians also experience street conditions themselves by riding in an ambulance as an observer. This is considered invaluable for anyone interested in obtaining first-hand knowledge. According to some paramedics at County, however, even this approach to understanding has its limitations, because when a doctor accompanies an ambulance crew and attempts to help, the work often does not go well. The doctor either interferes with the work of the paramedics or attempts to introduce medical techniques that physicians are capable of doing but that are considered inappropriate to the kind of care paramedics are mandated to give.

Vince, a County paramedic on the day-shift addressed the latter problem in this way:

> Well, we've had Dr. Anderson along a few times, but things don't go smoothly when he rides. He doesn't understand the street! Once he gave a patient a pelvic exam for God's sake. Now we can't do that.

Eric, another County paramedic, also expressed his view of having doctors as observers:

> Doctors are used to working in the controlled environment of the emergency room. There's plenty of help available, sterile condition, and all the supplies they need. But on the street everything is different, and they don't seem to realize this. I'll tell you when doctors go along on a run, the best thing they can do is to direct traffic and stay out of our way!

Sometimes the problem of the division of authority between paramedic and physician can become more confrontational. This frequently occurs when paramedics on the scene are attempting to provide advanced life support to a patient, and the doctor who is there as observer and has no official capacity, nonetheless attempts to intervene by asserting his or her authority. In such cases, paramedics cannot prevent the medical intrusion of the physician, since any licensed M.D. represents higher authority. On the other hand, unless the physician in question is well skilled and versed in emergency medicine, County paramedics consider the intervention as an unwarranted and unnecessary intrusion. Several paramedics at County had such examples to relate. In a sense, all took the form of atrocity stories. The following single incident should suffice:

> *Rodney (a night-shift paramedic):* We had a run to the baseball stadium—a guy had a cardiac arrest right in the stands. We went to work on him, and there was a crowd watching us. After a few minutes, a man pushed through the crowd and introduced himself as an intern. He started to examine our patient, and was getting in our way. I was doing an airway, and I had laid out my instruments getting ready to intubate the patient. When I reached around to get one of my instruments, it was gone! Later I discovered this intern had it. I asked him why he took it, and he said, "You don't think I was going to let you tube him, do you?"

Rodney in a later conversation asserted that he did not object to doctors offering help at the scene if they were conversant with emergency medical procedure:

> We get some doctors who will come up to us at the scene and say, "I'm a doctor, but I'm not up on a case like this—but I'll help however I can." Now that's the kind of doctors you like to get. Some of them though, just get in the way. But when we ask them [the doctors] if they want to assume medical authority, they'll disappear into the woodwork!

Despite these problems, paramedics often develop close relationships with emergency-room physicians, and these relationships often assume the qualities of a teacher-learner model. A number of paramedics at County Hospital while I was there seemed anxious to learn as much as they could about medical diagnosis and procedure. They appeared to have a strong identification with the more established health-care professionals and to seek out opportunities to put themselves in a learning situation.

Some emergency-room physicians are held in high esteem by paramedics, not only because they are willing to give appropriate field orders but also because they are willing to give informal advice and instruction in the hospital emergency room.

Such instructions may take several forms—from informal shoptalk about medical procedures and techniques to the more formal arrangements of in-service seminars to workshops on emergency care, taught by noted authorities in a particular field. Paramedics consider the in-service classroom sessions to be of some value, although they are not thought to be as important as those learning opportunities involving direct practical personal experience. It was for this reason that many of the paramedics observed in Metro-City used the emergency room at Mercy Hospital when the choice was within their discretion. According to these paramedics, the Mercy emergency-room doctors were not only among the most willing to give field orders, but also the most willing to give paramedics opportunities for direct "hands-on" experience in emergency-care procedures.

Many of the procedures that paramedics are expected to perform, such as inserting an "endotracheal" tube down a patient's throat, are quite difficult to do correctly and require much practice and experience. For the newer paramedics such practical experience is eagerly sought, and on occasion the physicians at Mercy allowed paramedics to practice inserting endotracheal tubes on patients who had died in the emergency room. Such procedures were not practiced on all dead patients, nor did all emergency-room physicians cooperate in these sessions. Nevertheless, however infrequent these learning situations might be, they occurred often enough for County paramedics to regard the emergency room at Mercy as more than a place to transport critically ill patients; it was a learning environment where valuable practice and experience might be obtained.

The following conversation between two County paramedics illustrates the importance of the "getting-practice" ideal:

> *Vince:* You know Dr. ——— at Mercy has really shown me a lot about intubation. I've really learned a lot from him.
>
> *Eric:* Yeah—I remember once we had a patient that we just couldn't get him tubed. He was dead by the time we got to Mercy. Dr. ——— showed us how to intubate the guy, and then he let each of us practice tubing him.
>
> *Researcher:* Is this fairly common over at Mercy?
>
> *Eric:* Oh, yeah. Hell, that's the way you learn to do things—they let us practice on people who have died in the emergency room.

Earlier in this chapter, it was mentioned that many paramedics at County Hospital had difficulty in obtaining field orders from some of the emergency-room doctors in Metro-City. While this can be a problem, some paramedics argued that the converse to that problem is the physician who gives too many orders, or who gives directives for procedures and techniques that paramedics feel go beyond what they are trained or legally mandated to do.

An experienced paramedic at County, who referred to such physicians as Super Docs, explained the nature of this problem:

> There is also Super Doc out there. And Super Doc wants you to do everything out there in the street that he would do in the hospital. Sometimes we get orders for things we shouldn't be doing! They're for us one hundred percent, but they are getting too far ahead of us. Either they're living dangerous, or they've got more confidence in us than we have in ourselves.

Although the paramedic quoted appreciated the support and confidence of emergency-room physicians, he apparently was aware of such a thing as "overordering." Paramedics often think of themselves as extensions of physicians, in carrying out certain medical directives at emergency scenes where doctors cannot be. It appears, however, that some paramedics have no desire to be surrogate physicians or to replace the doctor at the scene. In their working relations with emergency-room physicians in Metro-City, County paramedics sought the kind of support, confidence, and cooperation that falls somewhere in the middle of a continuum between those doctors who will not issue orders for "patients they can't see" and those "Super Docs" who expect paramedics to assume the role of physician-surrogate.

SUMMARY

While the cooperative aspects of medical care are coming to the attention of investigators interested in the importance of the team approach to emergency patient care, the fact remains that the traditional medical professions—medicine and nursing—are still highly individualized occupations. While nurses and doctors cooperate with each other in coordinating patient care, neither nurses nor physicians customarily work in partnership. For the EMT and paramedic, excessive individualism is almost always considered inappropriate.

In defining the qualities of a good EMT or paramedic, the men and women in the ambulance division of County Hospital virtually always stressed the importance of trust, cooperation, and willingness to share and to be relied on. Above all else, the "good" EMT or paramedic can be counted on as a partner. Where a person received his or her training, his or her degree of experience, proficiency in emergency techniques and skills, are always considered secondary in importance to the person's ability to work as a partner.

In this sense, while paramedics and EMTs at County saw themselves as budding health-care professionals, their work had much in common with other street emergency workers, i.e., the police and firemen, who also work in partnerships and crews. To work in the streets, whether to uphold law and order, extinguish fires, or deliver emergency medical care is to share the common circumstance that individual personal actions and motives count for very little. Whatever the branch of work, the dangers, risks, and uncertainties demand the sustained and coordinated action of crews and partners. No matter how proficient, knowledgeable, and competent such workers may be, they are only as good as their partner or crew. Whatever rewards and triumphs, failures and tribulations, come as a result of the work are never accepted alone or individually. They are part of the shared arrangements that characterize the work of police, firemen, and ambulance EMTs and paramedics. While the paramedics and EMTs at County Hospital often viewed the police and firemen as their rivals in emergency care, few would refuse to acknowledge that all three share in common the need to seek and create the kind of trust and mutual reliance that can spell the difference among coworkers between not only successful and unsuccessful emergency outcomes, but the difference between personal safety and security and peril.

Perhaps one of the most intriguing sociological features of emergency ambulance crews, both paramedic and EMT, is that while they share much in common and must learn to work on the scene with fellow emergency workers, theirs is also the world of the hospital from which they are dispatched and to which they transport their patients. In working on an everyday basis with doctors and nurses, a good part of the occupational identification of the EMTs and paramedics at County Hospital was with the men and women in white. In this sense, emergency ambulance work straddles two worlds: the street and the hospital.

Paramedics and EMTs need and seek the support and approval of the doctors and nurses with whom they work for two reasons. In the first place, there is no way in which emergency ambulance work can be conducted without a cooperative working relationship with emergency-room doctors and nurses. Where otherwise would EMTs and paramedics transport their patients? Secondly, as an emerging health-care profession, EMTs and paramedics depend upon doctors and nurses as role models and instructors, and as allies in their struggle for recognition as deserving professionals in the world of health-care work. Inasmuch as the role of emergency ambulance work is only possible because the medical profession bestows its blessing, the future importance of EMTs and paramedics depends on the continual support and encouragement of the physician.

Each time a patient is transported to an emergency-room facility is more than an occasion to display the techniques of prehospital emergency medicine; it is an opportunity to demonstrate to two important medical groups—doctors and nurses—the capabilities and potentials of the role of EMT and paramedic. As the EMT and paramedic places himself or herself in a position to learn from an emergency-room doctor something more about medical emergency technique, it provides the doctor with an opportunity not only to teach but also to give approval and recognition.

5

EMT AND PARAMEDIC VALUES AND ATTITUDES TOWARD THEIR WORK

No study of any occupational group is complete without a description of the values and attitudes such people hold toward their work. To pursue an occupation is more than making a living and carrying out a given round of daily activities. People also think about the work they do; they want it to have value and meaning for them. They think about what they like and dislike about it, what it is all about, what makes it worth doing. The meaning of work also includes the rewards of satisfactory work performance, not just the economic reward, but the psychic reward as well. If an occupation requires some degree of training and education, and involves serving a specific clientele, the meaning of the work will also have to do with ideas about how the clientele should be served, and consideration of what constitutes legitimate client demands and behavior, plus the different kinds of values placed on the outcomes of the client-provider relationship. People who work in human-service occupations are concerned with both the content of their work and the quantity and quality of the outcome that results from their efforts.

The paramedics and EMTs who worked in the emergency ambulance crews in Metro-City had their own attitudes and values about their work. Virtually every aspect of their daily routine was permeated by some value or attitude that made the work meaningful and important. Like all human-service workers, much of their work was defined in terms of their clientele—the patients whom they served, and, of course, in terms of the demands placed upon them by the patients and the circumstances in which the patients found themselves.

To explore the world of the emergency ambulance crew is to learn something about how the paramedics and EMTs see themselves, their work, their patients, and the larger community arena in which their professional activities are carried out. In fact, however, all these elements are interrelated. Paramedics and EMTs cannot consider themselves except in relation to their patients, and their work is, in a sense, the embodiment of that relationship. Moreover, the community milieu shapes their work in many ways and contributes to the ultimate boundaries of their world. If then we are to understand something of the nature of paramedic and EMT work, we must pay attention to how they view themselves, the people they treat, and the very unique and special demands that go with the job of performing emergency medicine in ambulances. Our exploration into the world of EMT and paramedic values begins with the emergency ambulance run and with what it represents in the larger scheme of work.

When an ambulance is dispatched to go to the service of an emergency victim, this process, as we have already seen, is referred to as a run. Responding to runs is considered to be the central duty and responsibility of EMTs and paramedics. For emergency ambulance crews, the run constitutes more than their occupational responsibility; it is their reason for working in the first place. The run is the beginning and the end of any thoughts and meanings given to their work. Nearly every other aspect of EMT and paramedic work is defined in terms of its effect on responding to a run. The run is what emergency ambulance work is all about; the skills acquired in training, the capacity to work smoothly and efficiently, the ability to keep one's cool in pressure-filled situations—these and other work considerations are important only insofar as they affect performance on a run.

When an EMT or paramedic reports for work at the beginning of a shift period, and his or her time card is punched, it does not mean that work has begun. In this sense he or she has only reported for duty; whether or not work will be forthcoming depends on how runs are alloted to particular crews. To be at work is in actuality only to be ready for work in terms of responding to a run. More important, for the individual paramedic or EMT, claims to skills, abilities, and capacities are valid only insofar as they are displayed during a run. No matter how skillful at emergency medical techniques, how efficient in patient care, how cool in emergency situations an EMT or paramedic may claim to be, unless he or she can prove it in responding on an emergency run, they are considered hollow claims. The measure of a man or woman doing EMT or paramedic work is always decided at the scene, not in the shoptalk of the crew room. Whatever boasting a person does to colleagues must always be backed up by behavior during a run, if it is to have any validity at all. The run is the ultimate determiner of one's capacity to do emergency work. "On paper" an EMT might be considered of high potential, because of intelligence, training, grades, and personality. But until that person shows at the scene what he or she is made of, it counts for very little. It is therefore worthwhile to examine the more general problem of runs and what they mean for EMTs and paramedics.

In an earlier chapter, the County Hospital ambulance division was described as having a dual-response system. This means quite simply that the district ambulance units, which are staffed by two EMTs, respond to only and all runs calling for basic life support. These runs cover the gamut from minor illnesses, injuries, and accidents, to the more serious situations that call for paramedic support. The paramedic units, which are staffed by two paramedics and by an EMT who acts as general assistant and driver, respond to life-threatening emergencies—the acutely ill, the traumatically injured. Although there are many exceptions, this means that the district ambulances get far more of the less serious runs, and the paramedic units a majority of the more critical cases. Of course, on most life-threatening emergencies a district ambulance is dispatched as well to act as an assistant crew for the paramedic unit.

Part, then, of the way in which emergency runs are evaluated by ambulance personnel has to do with preferences for working exclusively with life-threatening emergencies or with mostly basic life-support situations. For the EMT who works mostly in basic life support, the decision to seek advanced training and promotion to paramedic status is in part weighed in terms of one's preference for basic or advanced life support. Each type of patient and situation is considered by EMTs and paramedics to have certain advantages and disadvantages. For example, it is thought that the district ambulances see a wide variety of patients and conditions. While most of the patients are neither acutely ill nor injured, they are serious enough to warrant calling an ambulance (exceptions to this will be discussed later), and their conditions cover a wide range of disorders, physical, emotional, and mental. Often the patient is conscious, capable of talking and describing his or her problems with the EMTs on the scene. In paramedic runs, on the other hand, the patient is not only in critical condition but often unconscious and incapable of responding. Such a paramedic must therefore be the sort of person who derives satisfaction from working with this kind of patient.

While paramedics get used to their work, just like anyone else, some of them regard the constant stream of such patients as occasionally less than satisfactory. One experienced paramedic expressed it this way:

Sometimes I wish I were still an EMT rather than a paramedic. They [EMTs] get more variety of cases, and they can get more personalized relationships with their patients. Often they aren't

badly hurt, and you can talk to them and have a more personal relationship. Hell, all we [paramedics] see are dead people. All of
them are critical—and they usually can't talk. For us every run is
tense because we don't see any light cases. They're all critical!

On the other hand, some EMTs think that much of their work is done
on cases that are not really serious enough to need the intervention of an
EMT. As we shall examine later, many EMTs feel that people use an ambulance merely as a means of transportation to the hospital for an appointment or of getting the attention that they have failed to receive from
others in their immediate environment. In such cases, district ambulance
crews often feel that they have been put upon by people who abuse the
ambulance service. An EMT driver on a paramedic ambulance expressed
these thoughts:

Researcher: Joan, why do you work as an EMT driver for a paramedic unit rather than work the districts?

Joan: I really don't like riding the districts because of all the bullshit you see in the district. You get so many people who have no
business calling an ambulance just because they want a ride to the
hospital. Especially the poor people.

Because responding to runs is considered to be the most important
thing that EMTs and paramedics do, and because so much of their
validation of occupational esteem and worth is demonstrated under
actual run conditions, all EMT and paramedic crews want their share of
them on a given shift of duty. Yet there seems to be a sort of critical
ratio of runs to "time-out." All runs involve a high level of tension, risk,
and danger, so that no crew wants more than its share of runs, because
it is felt that no crew can work well at the scene if they are exhausted;
yet at the same time, no crew wants too few runs so that everyone becomes bored and tense waiting for something to happen. Having things
too quiet with few runs can sometimes be just as filled with strain as
having too many.

My own observations seem to indicate that at County Hospital each
crew wanted enough runs to "keep busy" but no more than their share
relative to the other ambulance units. In this sense, being busy or having
a slow shift was normally defined in relationship to the other crews in
Metro-City as well as in relationship to other similar shifts, the time of
day, of year, and so forth. Each crew, then, had an idea of the number
of runs it was taking relative to all the other crews. While some districts
of Metro-City were busier than others, it often occurred that one of the
ambulance units had to be out of service temporarily because of mechanical difficulties, or to obtain supplies, or for some other similar reason.
On such occasions, another crew would cover for that unit's runs, which

meant that the other ambulance unit would have two districts to cover. If it was a particularly slow shift, such additional coverage might be considered welcome because it doubled the opportunity to receive a run from dispatch communications. On the other hand, if it happened to be an especially busy shift, a crew that was responding to another district's calls might not find it desirable. The following interchange took place while I was present as an observer:

> While riding Paramedic I today, we responded to two runs that should have been covered by Medic II, since the runs were in their district. Both times, Medic II was temporarily out of service. The second time it happened we were just going to get some lunch when dispatch gave out the run. While we were proceeding to the scene, Vera, one of the paramedics in the crew who was sitting in the rear compartment with me, yelled (to be heard over the siren's noise) to the front seat to Vic, the other paramedic, "Where in the hell is Medic II? This should be their run!" Vic replied, "I don't know. They haven't taken a fucking run all day!"

In the above example both Vera and Vic felt that Paramedic Unit II was finding ways of staying out of service, which necessitated that their own crew handle more runs than they considered fair—though there was little that they could do about the situation other than hope that they would soon get some relief.

Aside from the distinction made in the ambulance division of County Hospital between basic life-support runs and advanced life-support or paramedic runs, there are other ways that runs are evaluated by EMTs and paramedics. Like all workers, paramedics and EMTs place certain values upon and give various meanings to the work they do. Although responding to runs is thought to be the most important aspect of their occupation, not all runs are thought to be equally valuable or to place legitimate demands upon their expertise.

In general, EMTs and paramedics are trained to respond to and act upon medical emergencies, some of which will be more severe than others. While, as we shall see, not all runs measure up, legitimate runs are thought to be those requiring emergency medical intervention, utilizing the training and skills of the EMT or paramedic. Emergency runs that fail to meet this basic requirement are considered to be illegitimate demands and negatively valued. Broadly speaking, emergency ambulance personnel want the kind of runs that permit them to put their emergency medical skills to use, and they consider as legitimate and worthwhile every run that meets that basic qualification. However, since no run can be refused by an ambulance unit, many runs are responded to that are considered illegitimate because there is virtually no opportunity for emergency medical intervention.

On a given tour of duty, an EMT or paramedic crew will have some legitimate good runs and some illegitimate bad runs, and the hope is that one will see more of the former than the latter. In this sense, paramedics and EMTs are similar in their occupational values to many other human-service providers, such as physicians, nurses, and social workers—to cite just a few—who think of their work largely in terms of the appropriate-ness of the demands placed upon them by their clientele. For such occupations, good and bad work experiences are largely thought of in terms of good and bad clientele, and the psychic rewards of work defined in some way relevant to the kinds of problems presented by clients. Among EMTs and paramedics, there are individual differences as to what kinds of runs a person likes to respond to, but there are also some more collective sentiments and values that appear to be shared by the whole collegial group.

GOOD RUNS

As stated earlier, for a run to be considered good, valuable, and legiti-mate the patient seeking help must require at least some degree of emer-gency medical intervention. The EMTs or paramedics who respond to the run must get some sense of having used their medical expertise in assist-ing the patient. While no run can be refused, this does not mean, as I have already indicated, that all runs produce the same level of satisfac-tion. Of course there are individual variations within the larger categories of legitimacy and value. For example while all paramedic crews want to respond to advanced life-support runs, some paramedics consider certain advanced life-support work more valuable or worthwhile than others.

Lewis, an experienced paramedic at County Hospital had spent much of his adult life working in ambulances and held strong opinions and attitudes about what kinds of runs he really valued:

> *Lewis:* I'll tell you honestly, I'm a trauma freak. Those are the kinds of runs I like to go on. I think trauma is much more challeng-ing than working on people in cardiac arrest. You know, in a cardiac arrest, there is only so much you can do for the patient. But in trauma there are endless possibilities of what to do or think about.
> *Researcher:* Does it bother you to see people badly hurt?
> *Lewis:* Hell, no—nothing bothers me anymore.

On another occasion while I was riding as an observer with a paramedic unit that included Lewis in the crew, we had just completed a run when the ambulance developed mechanical problems. As a result we had to be temporarily out of service until the vehicle could be repaired. While our unit was out of service, the dispatcher gave out a run for Code 12 to the other paramedic unit that was covering the district with us. When Lewis heard the dispatcher give out the run, he remarked, "Damn it, here we are ten-seven [out of service], and we've missed a Code Twelve."

The collective sentiments are what is of interest here, and it should be instructive now to look more closely at the various categories of runs that are considered good runs by virtually every County Hospital EMT and paramedic. All these runs are defined as having positive values for those doing emergency ambulance work. They are the runs that produce approval, confidence, and on some occasions, even elation. They are the kinds of emergency runs pointed to with pride in the crew room, and in which everyone wants to be a part. The first category of positively valued runs I have termed "celebrated cases."

CELEBRATED CASES

Because EMT and paramedic crews work out in the open, there are occasions when what they do come to the attention of the larger public community. Usually this happens when the news media, especially the press and television, gives coverage to some important emergency disaster. Spectacular automobile accidents, homicides, large fires, explosions, airplane crashes, are all events to which the media gives broad coverage, and in so doing creates an important public happening. The reading or viewing public appears to be fascinated with disaster; the more spectacular, the better. For those who do rescue work—policemen, firemen, EMTs and paramedics—an emergency scene that is thoroughly covered by the media affords the opportunity to have their skills and expertise demonstrated to a wider audience than is usually the case. While the news media can at times get in the way, more often than not, it captures for the wider public some of the drama, excitement, and danger of those who do emergency work. While the police and firemen have had such favorable publicity for years, it is especially important to paramedics and EMTs who are trying to gain greater and more favorable public support for the work they do.

For the individual paramedic or EMT at County Hospital, the celebrated case was always considered worthwhile to be "in on" as it not only brought publicity to the ambulance division, but a kind of personal recognition that otherwise is rare in emergency ambulance work. To do

one's job well is important; to do it well at the scene of a highly publicized community emergency which draws the attention of many is all
the more significant and rewarding. The paramedics and EMTs at County
Hospital were sensitive to their public image (the ambulance division
employed a person to deal with public relations), and they were aware
of those occasions when runs in which they participated were reported
in the press and on television.

While almost all the EMTs and paramedics at County Hospital have
had their pictures appear in the media at least once, being on a crew that
responds to a highly publicized emergency defines the truly celebrated
case. In such an event, the occasion is not only celebrated, but all those
who have participated in it, bask in a sense, in the glory. The following
incident serves as an example:

> I was sitting in the crew room at one of the Metro-City hospitals
> during shift change. The day crew [paramedic] was going off-
> duty as the second shift was coming on. Vic, one of the second-
> shift paramedics, had just entered the crew room when one of the
> day-shift paramedics asked him about the events of the night before.
> This run had made front-page headlines and widespread TV cover-
> age—and continued to do so for several days. A man had entered
> a university medical laboratory with a rifle, shot an employee, and
> in so doing, set off a dramatic, fiery explosion in the university
> medical center.
>
> *Vic:* We [Paramedic Unit I] were the first emergency crew to get
> there since it was so close to the hospital. I was working with Lewis.
> We got there right after the explosion, and there was so much heat
> and smoke you couldn't see. Lewis yelled to Control that we would
> need air packs to get in.
>
> *Paramedic:* Why the hell did Lewis get so excited?
>
> *Vic:* I don't know. He just blew his cool. But later he admitted it.
> The firemen arrived pretty soon, and they went in to fight the fire.
> We kind of helped them by taking their temperatures when they
> would come out. I told the chief that he better let us tell the fire-
> men when to sit down—or they would have a fatality on their
> hands. And the chief agreed.
>
> *Paramedic:* Was the employee dead by the time you could get
> into the building?
>
> *Vic:* Yes. By the time Lewis and I could get in, the body was just
> boiled. It was really bad. If we could have got right in, I think we
> could have had a save. But there was no way we could get in. I ran
> all over trying to find a way in, but just couldn't.

The above dialogue shows the importance of the event not only for

Vic himself but for the second-shift ambulance crew as a whole. The crew gained recognition for being part of the rescue workers of a notable community emergency, one that continued to dominate the news media for several weeks. It contained all the essential ingredients for community drama: a million-dollar explosion and fire, death by violence, and the subsequent suicide attempt of the assailant. The media devoted close-up coverage to the attempts of the emergency workers (paramedics, firemen, and police) to subdue the fire and rescue any victim. For Vic, an experienced paramedic, and a person held in high regard by his colleagues, it afforded the opportunity to provide an insider's information about the run. Such runs, one does not get everyday, maybe even only once a year.

Vic and Lewis were first on the scene of what was to become one of the most talked-about and investigated community events in Metro-City. While Vic and Lewis were unable to save the gunshot victim, their work that day was worthwhile to them by the very fact of their being there, by being first on the scene, and working with other rescue workers in a common effort that the community regarded as important. For his colleagues in the crew room, Vic relived the emergency event, supplying details, which at that time few other people were privy to. There was a sense of satisfaction in the fact that it was his run, his crew, that was there first. His fellow paramedics that afternoon in the crew room shared the importance of the occasion, because they knew the impact that the whole affair had on Metro-City. And while the first-shift crew was not on the scene, someone they worked with, knew, and trusted was there, and in a certain sense they too could feel better about their work and mission.

SAVES

A second category of positively valued runs has already been introduced earlier when their importance was discussed. At that time "saves" were presented in the context that inasmuch as paramedics must confront on a daily basis the dangers and risks of ambulance work, it is the special contingencies of aiding dying or critically injured or ill patients that makes everything else seem somehow worthwhile. It is the saves that give paramedics and EMTs a reason for going on, for continuing their work, in spite of all the death and dying they so often confront. In the following section we shall examine the phenomenon of saves a little more closely.

A good deal of attention in recent years has been directed toward the development of an EMS (emergency medical services) system in the United States. Part of the function of such a system would be devoted to providing better-trained and -qualified ambulance personnel, so that inroads could be made in reducing the number of deaths from accidents and prehospital coronaries. According to the American College of Emergency Physicians, literally thousands of such deaths are preventable with improved prehospital emergency care. As we saw in Chapter 1, this national attention has meant a significant upgrading in the training and education of ambulance personnel in the United States in general; at County Hospital, for example, no persons can work in the ambulance crew without EMT certification. The paramedics receive some of the most advanced and sophisticated training to be found in the field of advanced life support. How successful the EMS system will be in reducing the number of preventable deaths remains to be seen. That is outside the scope of this discussion. Our present purpose is to examine this advanced training from the point of view of the paramedic.

Paramedics acquire a sense of confidence in their abilities to help emergency victims as they go through their training and gain street experience. In part, the nature of their work demands a certain level of self-confidence and belief in their abilities. Paramedics look forward to challenging emergency situations in which their skills are tested. Implicit in their training, their public and media image, their reputation in the world of emergency workers, is the idea that paramedics save lives; i.e., by applying the techniques of advanced life support, they prevent the deaths of accident and coronary victims and others who otherwise might not live to reach a hospital. In this sense, saving a life is not only something that makes the job rewarding and worthwhile and is a way of coping with the stress of the work; it is also something that paramedics routinely expect to do. It is expected in the sense that periodically in the course of casual conversation paramedics will assess the number of saves recently accomplished, the near misses, and of course, the failures. In reality the failures far outnumber the near misses and the successes.

Every paramedic knows that saves are few and far between, and while the rookie may keep an accurate count of the number in which he or she has participated, the experienced paramedic no longer does so. In fact, this is one of the distinguishing features between the rookie and the seasoned paramedic: the seasoned worker has lost track of his or her significant runs. For the experienced paramedic, it is not so much that the number of saves is so overwhelming; it is just that it no longer seems important to keep count of them. Nevertheless, even for the experienced paramedic, each save has a positive value and serves as a highlight for the day or week in which it occurs, depending on the number of saves accomplished.

The definition of what constitutes a save is less easy to describe since there is some variation among paramedics of what a save actually is. The most general description would include keeping someone who is facing immediate death from accident or illness alive long enough to be admitted to a hospital ward. Since paramedics also have a difficult time agreeing on a definition of immediate death, this general description is usually not used. My own observations revealed that when the paramedics at County Hospital talked above saves they referred to people, usually coronary victims, whose vital signs—pulse, blood pressure, respiration—indicated death and who were then resuscitated. In an earlier era of ambulance care, such a victim would nearly always have been dead on arrival. There also seems to be some disagreement as to how long the victim must remain alive following resuscitation.

For some paramedics at County, a save was any successful resuscitation of a coronary victim who lives long enough to be admitted to a ward in the hospital. For other paramedics the patient must eventually live long enough to leave the hospital. Eric, an experienced paramedic with many years on the squad, held to the latter definition:

> *Eric:* To me a save means somebody is resuscitated and lives through the hospital and is alive six months later. To me that's a good save.
> *Researcher:* How do you know they are alive six months later?
> *Eric:* Well, we used to do our own follow-up on a patient. I don't do it anymore though.
> *Researcher:* Could you give me an example of what for you is a good save?
> *Eric:* We had one the other day that was unbelievable. This guy was seventy-three years old and had just flown in from the East, and was walking through the airport—and he went into cardiac arrest. Security personnel at the airport started CPR. When we got there, Car Five [the shift supervisor] was already there, and he had started an IV on the guy and had pushed some drugs. And it just happened that there was an M.D. who walked up on the scene, and she defibrillated the patient. When we got there, the guy had his own heart rate, pulse, and blood pressure. By the time we got him to County, I was talking to him about Puerto Rico— that's where he was going. To me that was great. There was no brain damage—nothing. You don't get many like that.

While there is some disagreement among paramedics as to how long the patient must live after resuscitation, there is general agreement that the patient must at least make it to the hospital emergency room and be a viable patient; i.e., one who has the potential to make a complete recovery. In this sense many paramedics make a distinction between a save and a resuscitation; they are not the same thing. A person can be resuscitated and still not be a viable patient.

Eric, the paramedic quoted above, also discussed this distinction: We can resuscitate a lot of people. Even if they've blown their brains out, we can keep their heart working. But they're not going anywhere. They'll [the hospital emergency room] take them upstairs and plant them like a carrot. But that's not a save. They'll just unplug them—and take their kidneys out or something. We resuscitate those people—like a suicide, or gunshot to the head— we resuscitate them, not because we think they'll be a save, but to get their kidneys. Maybe they can be a donor. We've had a lot of those.

It seems to be the case that while every paramedic expects to accomplish a number of saves in his or her career, they do not come easy or often. When they do happen, it can serve to revitalize a crew and give them some good moments; it is something to be proud of, something to share in the shoptalk of the crew room. However as we have already seen and as is all too often the case, saves occur with no predictability. Paramedics, it must be reiterated, live in an uncertain world. County Hospital paramedics admitted to me that they might go for weeks without a single save and then get two in one morning—such is the nature of the work. While each paramedic crew may do all they can for a patient in cardiac arrest, statistics demonstrate that the odds are far from favorable. For every successful resuscitation, there are a great many patients who never get to a hospital emergency room, or if they do, never leave it alive.

In that sense, the elusive thing about a save is that to achieve one, as paramedics define it, the patient must virtually be dead—in which case the probabilities of success are indeed very slight. For some paramedics the whole phenomenon of the save can be a source of frustration as well as reward. Because most victims of coronary arrest do not live, paramedics look at the characteristics of the patient to give them a clue of their chances to obtain a save. In general terms, they expect, for example, that the younger the victim is, the greater is the chance for success. Conversely, the elderly patient in full cardiac arrest is worked on, but with less expectation of a rewarding outcome. Even this distinction, however, cannot always be relied upon as the forces of life and death, over which paramedics have no control, often disregard this kind of medical logic. Alan, a County Hospital paramedic of several years' experience, marched into the administrative offices of the ambulance division one morning and vented his feelings of frustration on the secretary:

Alan: I don't know what the hell to think anymore.

Secretary: Why, what's the matter?

Alan: Hell, I can't save anyone anymore! We lost a twenty-eight-year-old, a forty-year-old, and today we saved a seventy-eight-year-old. Now what the shit's going on?

For Alan, things just had not worked out as expected as far as his saves were concerned. Subsequent conversation with him revealed that he did not object to the seventy-eight-year-old patient making it, but that he was at a loss to explain why he and his partner had been unable to save the younger victims. In Alan's view, this was what the work was all about; and when it is the younger patients who die, that fact challenges what little certainty paramedics are able to structure into their work. The fact that Alan expected to achieve a save on the younger patients further substantiates our earlier argument, that while saves do not occur very often, every paramedic expects to achieve some, and when the patient is young, it increases the sense of expectation.

One County Hospital paramedic, George, went so far as to request from the ambulance division that he be allowed to see the coroner's report on a twenty-eight-year-old medical student whom he and his crew had vainly attempted to resuscitate. For George, the victim's youth and background as a medical student made him such a likelihood for a save that when he and his partner failed, he almost could not believe it. George's later request to see a copy of the coroner's report was his way of dealing with his sense of futility, hoping to find in the report some aspect of the patient's physical condition about which he and his partner had been unaware.

Despite the fact that saves are not always accomplished when paramedics expect them to be, a run that results in a save is still the most highly and positively valued one. For County paramedics with several years of experience in the ambulance division, it was the one event that kept them working and made them change their minds when they were thinking about switching careers. A save is exceedingly important, not because it happens relatively infrequently, but because it happens at all. It comes close to one of the most fundamental human values found in society—the act of risking one's own safety and comfort to save another person's life. While paramedics do this as part of their occupational obligation and routine, it is no less meaningful to them. In this sense, the meaning of the save is lifted out of its occupational context, and stands as something more profound than simply doing one's job correctly. And although on the one hand it is ironic that such occasions do not happen more frequently, on the other, for most paramedics there is deep satisfaction that they occur at all.

LEARNING EXPERIENCE

Throughout this book the idea of street experience has been referred to repeatedly. Basically, it means that EMTs and paramedics learn how to do their work and to be of help to emergency patients in two ways. They learn from the formal classroom training, which they receive before they are certified for work in an emergency ambulance. This part of their training, which is conducted by physicians, nurses, and EMT educators, includes textbook materials, films, written work, and various other activities that take place in a formal classroom setting. The second kind of educational training is derived from experience gained on the job. This includes what is learned from listening to shoptalk in the crew room, the advice given by senior colleagues, and the various experiences that are generated from working with emergency patients.

Earlier we saw that for many if not most EMTs and paramedics the formal classroom training they receive prepares them in only a general way for their actual work. Much of what they learn that will be of use to patients must be learned in the street. The classroom experience, while important, cannot anticipate all the special circumstances that EMTs and paramedics must confront, and most of them soon discover that much of what they can do for patients will be situationally mandated. In short, no two patients or emergency situations are exactly alike, and for an EMT or paramedic to work effectively, it is generally felt that the more situations and patients confronted, the better able he or she will be to make sound medical judgments. Street experience then becomes a matter of paramount value in the world of the EMT and paramedic.

In this light, all the runs that are participated in have an intrinsic importance, since they provide experience; and in a most basic way, the more runs one has experienced the better, because almost always something is learned. However, the EMTs and paramedics at County Hospital felt that some runs were more important than others because of their learning potential. In more general terms, unusual cases are highly valued because they are not confronted routinely. An emergency victim with an unusual injury or illness provides valuable experience, primarily because the case is unusual, not one typically confronted. Likewise emergency runs that require the utilization of a high degree of skill are also highly valued.

The classroom dimension of EMT training is basically training in the

skills of emergency care. For paramedics, it includes some highly sophisticated and complex medical diagnostic procedures, such as intravenous
cannulation, endotracheal intubation, recognition of cardiac arrhythmias,
and intravenous administration of drugs. These skills, once acquired,
must be called upon often enough for a paramedic to retain competency,
let alone mastery. Therefore all emergency ambulance runs that require
utilization of some or all of the skills fit high into the value hierarchy.
A good run is, above all else, one that will call for the EMT and paramedic to call upon his or her training in using crucial medical and diagnostic procedures. It is this that produces a high sense of satisfaction
and accomplishment. As we shall see a bit later in this chapter, a good
many of the runs that paramedics and EMTs go on fail to satisfy the above
requirements and thus become negatively valued and a source of
annoyance.

It is difficult if not impossible to construct a typology of cases that
result in learning experience. Obviously, a rookie paramedic will look
upon each run as more valuable than will a veteran, since each case
represents something new and an opportunity to put newly acquired
skills and techniques to use. However, some examples of the kind of run
that seemed to represent for the EMTs and paramedics involved, some
aspects of the experiential type of learning will now be presented.

Richard, an EMT at County Hospital, had been employed in the ambulance division for almost a year. Prior to that, he had worked a year for
a private ambulance company in Metro-City, making mostly convalescent
transfers. He told me that on his first day of work for County he saw
the worst automobile wreck of his career. It happened while he was off-
duty, driving home. On the Interstate he came upon an accident that had
just occurred, the dust from the wreck was still settling.

Richard was the first person on the scene. He got out the tech box
he carried in the trunk of his car and examined the wreck. The cars involved were totally demolished, and the first three occupants of the cars
he examined were dead. One female passenger, Richard determined, was
alive but with her chest crushed. He administered some first aid to her.
In the meantime, a fire department rescue truck appeared on the scene,
and Richard called for them to bring some shock pants for the female
patient.

Richard thought he had seen all the victims and was preparing to
turn things over to the fire department rescue truck when he heard
screaming from the rear of one of the cars. Richard dug through luggage
and other material compacted in the rear compartment and found a
young boy pinned under the rear seat. The boy had a fractured arm,

and it took some time for the firemen to remove the patient from the car.

For Richard the accident represented a learning experience which was significant to him for several reasons. First, while this was not a legitimate run, since he was off duty, it was a situation that put him on the spot as an EMT. It called for him to act as a first responder to a severe medical emergency, to evaluate the scene, to maintain his cool, and to do some of the things he was trained to do. Richard admitted that it was a difficult undertaking because the cars involved were so wholly demolished, and the first three people he examined were not only dead but the victims of severe crushing injuries. In short, it was a gross, unpleasant, and totally dismaying scene, yet one that provided for him a glimpse, on his first day of work, of what his occupational life would now be filled. Not that he would see such tragedy everyday, but that these would certainly not be the last deaths by violence he would face in the years to come. The accident also gave Richard an opportunity to see how he would handle himself in such a situation. It represented for him a test of his ability as an EMT to rise to the occasion and prove something to himself. It was the kind of learning experience that not all EMTs receive, since it occurred so early in his career and when he was alone. Richard confided that he learned not only something about the treatment of traumatic injuries at an accident site but something about his own emotional reactions and responses to seeing this sort of dying and mutilation.

There is another category of emergency run that can provide EMTs and paramedics with an invaluable learning experience, and this includes those runs in which the patient has an unusual medical condition that stimulates the thinking and curiosity of the emergency ambulance staff involved.

Many of the paramedics and EMTs at County Hospital were interested in medicine and disease from an intellectual standpoint. Their concerns went beyond the limited application of emergency techniques and skills, and extended into an intellectual desire to know what caused a patient's condition, i.e., why the patient died or became ill. For EMTs and paramedics with this orientation, a positively valued run is one in which they learn something about disease, physiology, anatomy. Usually this involves the paramedics who took the run asking the doctor in the emergency room about the patient's condition when they bring the patient in. In many cases, paramedics will follow the progress of a patient to see the outcome of the injury or illness as a way of discovering more about pathological consequences. The following incident will serve as an illustration:

One of the paramedic units was transporting a patient in serious condition to St. Regis Hospital. While en route the paramedics on duty, Dale and William, were in radio contact with an emergency-room physician who gave them several orders to administer drugs to the patient in the ambulance. Later in the morning, several hours after the patient was delivered to the emergency room and the paramedic crew had returned to County, Dale was preparing to call St. Regis Hospital to check on the condition of the patient. I wanted to find out the reasons for his call.

Researcher: Do you want to find out how he is doing, Dale?

Dale: I know how he is. I'm sure he's D.E.D. [dead]. I want to find out what was wrong. I think the guy might have had a pneumothorax, but I'm not sure.

After Dale had made the phone call, he returned to the crew room and announced to his partners: "Would you guys believe that the guy we took to St. Regis had a bilateral pneumothorax? I just called and that's what they said."

For Dale, that early morning was important as a learning occasion. While the outcome was unsuccessful, for the patient died, his condition was unusual enough to cause Dale to explore the pathological condition of the victim. Dale was a paramedic whose interest went beyond application of technique; he had to know why the patient died. His curiosity was aroused, and he had to satisfy it in an intellectually meaningful way. When his suspicion of a pneumothorax was confirmed, he was able to convince himself that although the patient had succumbed, the run had taught him something more about the human body. And, having learned that, he felt that he in some small way was now a more learned paramedic and had gained from the experience. It was Dale's way—and he was not alone in this among the County Hospital paramedics—of obtaining some satisfaction from an otherwise unsuccessful run.

The final category of positively valued runs is a very broad one and includes all those that call for EMTs and paramedics alike to use their skills and training on what they consider to be bona fide medical emergencies. For paramedics, this means that the patient must require at least some measure of advanced life support, and for EMTs it means that the patient has need of basic life support. In the section that follows, we will discuss those categories of runs that represent illegitimate demands for emergency medical service and are thus negatively valued.

I refer to the category of legitimate demands for emergency care as mission relevant. As I stated at the beginning of this chapter, all those who work in human-service occupations develop conceptions about what are appropriate and inappropriate requests for service. Because the roles of the EMT and paramedic are of recent development, emergency ambulance workers are conscious of what their work is and should be about. Having subjected themselves to the rigors of classroom training, they now want legitimate opportunities to use their skills on patients who need their help.

For a run to be considered appropriate or mission relevant, the patient need not necessarily be acutely ill or injured—although for a paramedic run this would normally be true. Many EMT runs, for example, involve patients who require an ambulance but are not in a life-or-death circumstance. The question is rather, Are EMT or paramedic skills called for? If some level of training and skill is required to handle the case, then it is mission relevant as far as the paramedic or EMT team is concerned. If it is something that the police or a member of the family could handle better, then it becomes an inappropriate request for aid. For example, many paramedic runs are made for victims of suspected coronaries. Often whoever phones Control describes a condition that indicates a heart problem, and the dispatcher allots the case to a paramedic crew. The paramedics often determine through various diagnostic procedures at the scene that the patient is not suffering a coronary. They may transport the patient—if the patient so requests—or they may turn the case over to a district ambulance crew. The point is that although the patient did not suffer a coronary, the run was appropriate because only after the paramedics' diagnostic skills had been used could that be determined. In this sense, while the patient was not in immediate danger, the emergency did require paramedic evaluation. In such a case, skills, both medical and diagnostic, were brought into play, and that fact legitimized the run.

Within this context it should be pointed out that while the run described above would have been defined as appropriate by most paramedics at County Hospital, it does not follow that such a run would be highly valued. Although a legitimate run and positively valued as relevant to the mission, it would not be considered as good a run as if it had been a real case of cardiac arrest. The more skills called for in helping a patient, the more positively valued for paramedics the run becomes.

Paramedics are trained in many complex techniques, and they feel that they need to employ these techniques fairly often if they are to retain their competency. While no paramedic crew wants a continuous stream of critical runs, they want enough to keep high their level of skill. Critical runs represent a broad spectrum of skill utilization then, and are accordingly prized. Interestingly, such considerations as location, time of day, and other factors are not of great importance. EMTs and paramedics become accustomed to the vicissitudes of street work. A run can be mission relevant even if it occurs under less than desirable conditions—at night, during a blizzard, at an explosion, and so forth. For the EMTs and paramedics who worked at County Hospital, the where, when, why, or how a patient needed medical assistance was not nearly so important as the condition of the patient. The important question becomes, To what degree does this request for emergency care involve the use of the training and skills that EMTs and paramedics are prepared to deliver? My own personal observations and interviews have indicated that this condition is paramount.

BAD RUNS

It was E. C. Hughes writing several years ago who called attention to the problems that all occupations face in doing work that goes counter to the norms of the occupation.[9] People who perform certain kinds of work attempt to control, as best they can, how they will perform the work activity. They develop conceptions of what is proper, dignified, and appropriate in work demands. Those who work in occupations that serve a clientele also develop definitions of what are legitimate demands for their service, and what are illegitimate demands and beyond the bounds of their service to provide. Professional services, in particular, attempt to control the context of their work through various means, but the most effective one is to restrict or be very selective in regard to clientele.

The paramedics and EMTs who work for County Hospital saw their work in the terms just described. They had ideas about what constituted an appropriate emergency request for help and what was an inappropriate one. They also performed a variety of occupational tasks which they found unpleasant and perhaps even undignified. I see these as two problematic features in emergency ambulance work. On the one hand, paramedics and EMTs want their work to contain a good share of medical heroics, yet their very occupation requires a variety of occupational duties that are neither heroic nor rewarding; in fact, these duties are often unpleasant and undignified. The problem for the EMT and paramedic is that there is little that can be done to avoid those runs that result in unpleasant, undignified, and unrewarding work. No run can be refused, and there is no occupation below the EMT in the emergency-care hierarchy to which these unsatisfactory tasks can be assigned. In short, it seems to be a situation that must be accepted and coped with, rather than changed.

The following discussion will be divided into two sections. First, we will examine the idea of "dirty work" as it applies to emergency ambulance workers; and second, we will look more closely at the various types of emergency runs that are considered to be illegitimate demands for service.

"Insofar as an occupation carries with it a self-conception, a notion of personal dignity, it is likely that at some point one will feel he is having to do something that is infra dignitate."[10] This quotation from Hughes highlights an important dimension in the analysis of any occupation. Every occupation will, no doubt, differ in terms of what it considers to be the undignified aspect of the work. And, of course, what is thought to be undignified in one occupation may be quite readily accepted in another.

For the EMTs and paramedics at County Hospital, their work, responding to medical emergencies, put them in a variety of situations in which they were exposed to dirty work. Not only did they work with the sick, the injured, the mutilated, the dying, and the dead, they worked on such patients in the most immediate sense. They confronted victims whose blood was still flowing, whose wounds were raw and exposed before anything had been done to clean up, apply sterile dressings, or make matters look better. In this respect, one result of what EMTs and paramedics do at the emergency scene is to make the emergency victim more presentable to the hospital emergency-room staff. By the time the emergency-room staff sees most patients, much of the dirt has been removed, the bleeding stopped, and sterilized white bandages and wrappings applied.

EMT and paramedic work is a "hands-on" activity in the strictest sense. Indeed emergency medical ambulance crews are among the very first persons actually to touch an emergency victim. In touching and handling the victim at the scene, before he or she can be cleaned up, bandaged, etc., and made to look more like a patient, the EMT and paramedic often come to share the victim's disarray. If the victim is dirty, bloody, smelly, or whatever, that condition is transferred to the care of the ambulance crew.

The dirty work of EMTs and paramedics is inherent in the two physical conditions under which they work. The first is the bodily physical condition of the emergency victims themselves—their wounds, sores, vomit, and so on. The second is the environmental physical condition of the emergency scene—slum, traffic accident, fire, explosion.

Every EMT and paramedic whom I talked with at County Hospital had his or her favorite dirty-work story—about handling a body that had been dead for several days, the stench of death, or the sight of maggots infesting the corpse. Almost all EMTs and paramedics argue that the smell of death is excruciatingly powerful, distasteful, one that lingers long after the encounter has ended.

In addition to having to work directly and immediately with victims who are often bloody, dirty, smelly, unwashed, or mutilated, there are also certain emergency techniques that paramedics and EMTs are called on to perform that are often considered distasteful. For example, mouth-to-mouth resuscitation is a technique necessary for aiding victims of coronary and respiratory arrest, as well as other accidents. Mouth-to-mouth resuscitation, while valuable, is considered most unpleasant by EMTs and paramedics if the victim has vomited or has unhygienic mouth and dental features. Some County Hospital EMTs and paramedics admitted that the technique was so unappealing that they did not perform it very often—if at all. According to Gus, one of the County EMTs:

> We don't like to use it very often because we get a lot of inner-city patients and you don't know what you will pick up.

Still another paramedic admitted that he had quit giving mouth-to-mouth resuscitation several years ago.

While some emergency techniques can be avoided, the fact remains that those first on the scene must handle the patient in a variety of conditions, and no EMT or paramedic can ever be assured that he or she will escape dirty work in the course of a given shift.

The second dimension of dirty work focuses on the conditions of the scene itself. Paramedics and EMTs are sent to many locations, a large number of which are thought to be less than desirable places to work. Some are dirty and noisy, such as industrial sites and scenes of traffic accidents. Others are physically uncomfortable, such as working in the open in the winter, exposed to wind, cold, and snow. Some sites are considered dangerous, such as slums, tenements, lower-class bars, and the like. Even the homes of victims are often rather unpleasant places in which to work.

Many ambulance runs that County EMTs and paramedics responded to were for inner-city residents whose homes and apartments were often dirty, noisy, cluttered, and crowded. For some County EMTs these home emergency scenes were among the most unpleasant in which to work. Alice had been working as an EMT for County about a year when she told me:

Many apartments we go into to treat patients, you wouldn't believe. Many have no heat, electricity, or plumbing. Some families in these apartments have jars they keep in the hallway to urinate in. When you go in at night, you have to be careful not to trip over them, because if you spill them, the smell is terrible.

Emergency ambulance crews must enter such buildings regardless of the conditions, however unpleasant they seem. Their work is to administer emergency medical care and transport the patient to the nearest hospital. No matter how shocking or miserable they may feel the living conditions of the victim to be, it must have no bearing on their work. Like the pain and suffering of the emergency patient, EMTs and paramedics must learn to "remove from consciousness" the immediate conditions of the scene. A description of a paramedic run, which I observed one afternoon, may provide an illustration:

The paramedic unit I was observing was given a run to the east side of Metro-City for an "unconscious patient." The address was a two-story frame home in which all the exterior paint was peeled off and several windows were broken and boarded up. We entered the living room, and several people were sitting in there. One teenage girl was holding a baby; there were two middle-age adults, and several young children running in and out of the house. Clothes were scattered throughout the room, cigarette butts covered much of the floor, as well as scraps of food and dirty dishes and paper plates. A small room off the living room contained a small unmade bed, and the entire room was littered with clothes, empty soft-drink cans, and newspapers.

The paramedic crew was directed upstairs, and at the top of the landing we turned into a room that was bare of any furniture or lighting fixtures. The walls were unpainted and contained but a few posters. One of the district crews was administering to a white male lying on the floor. He was nude except for his undershorts, and appeared to be around twenty years old, with a beard and crew-cut. He was unconscious and one of the district EMTs announced to us that the patient was having a grand-mal seizure. His body was rigid, eyes rolled back in his head, frothing at the mouth with spittle flying everywhere. He was making loud, gurgling noises that could be heard when we entered the building.

I surveyed the bathroom adjacent to the room the patient was in and found the plumbing fixtures broken, and broken glass and old magazines completely covering the bathroom floor. The patient's brother told the paramedics that the patient didn't live here, but came so he could be alone to "do drugs."

Such a scene is encountered virtually daily by EMTs and paramedics as they do their work. They often find their patients and carry out their duties in the dark, dingy, poverty-stricken conditions under which many people live and all too often die.

ILLEGITIMATE RUNS

Having looked at those runs that are considered legitimate demands for emergency ambulance service, it is important to underline that not all such runs are considered good. A run can be considered bad, i.e., unrewarding, because it is dirty, undignified, or requires few emergency medical skills or abilities, but every run is still considered a legitimate request for an emergency ambulance. There is, however, another category of runs, which EMTs and paramedics must embark upon, that are defined as inappropriate or illegitimate requests for aid. Every EMT and paramedic crew gets some of these runs, and since they cannot be avoided, they must somehow be endured. My personal observations and research indicate that this category constitutes the smallest number of runs, but since such runs create a sense of frustration in ambulance personnel, they must be included in our discussion.

Illegitimate runs fall into three subcategories, according to the EMTs and paramedics at County Hospital: crock runs, house calls, and taxi-service runs. Each type constitutes a special problematic feature of ambulance work, although as we shall see, there are common features among all three.

CROCK RUNS

The idea of the "crock" in the field of medical care does not originate with emergency ambulance workers. Among the first studies to report the use of the word among medical professionals was Howard S. Becker and his associates, in an early study of medical school socialization.[11] Becker discovered that medical students used the term to designate those hospital patients who complained of feeling poorly, but for whom no definable disease or injury can be discovered. Crock patients were considered to be a nuisance among medical students since there was no pathology the student could act upon yet the patient continued to play the sick role. In short, the crock patient had unfounded complaints.

The EMTs and paramedics at County Hospital encountered similar situations, in which they were called out on an emergency run when there was no emergency—at least no emergency as they defined one. In a sense, for ambulance work, the crock run comes close to the false alarm faced by firemen. Indeed, a crock run is often designated as one when an emergency ambulance is requested but the caller knows full well there is no medical emergency. In this way, whoever is phoning into dispatch Control for an ambulance is often trying to get the attention of some public authority to help with a problem, and since ambulances and fire departments always respond, they are among the first to be called. In fact, one of the clues the County Hospital paramedics used to anticipate a crock run, en route to the scene, was whether or not the fire department had been called to the scene without a fire having been reported. The following emergency run occurred one afternoon, while I was riding as an observer:

Our unit, Paramedic Unit I, was given a run by the dispatcher for an OD [drug overdose]. While we were en route, the dispatcher informed the crew that we would be joined at the scene by the Metro-City fire department. The dispatcher said that the fire department had a call from a box near the apartment where we were going. Eric, who was sitting in the rear of the ambulance with me, yelled out, "I think this may be a crock run."

We arrived at the address, a three-story walk-up apartment building, along with two fire trucks. Eric and the other paramedic, George, and our EMT driver, Vera, followed several firemen into the building. The firemen were all dressed in fire-fighting gear, complete with axes and extinguishers.

On the third floor, Eric and two firemen entered an apartment where several young black women sat in the living room. One of the women pointed to another young woman, and said, "Her boyfriend beat her up this morning." The young woman didn't request any medical attention, and Eric and George withdrew from the living room, as one of the fire officials talked to the woman about her boyfriend.

As we returned to the ambulance, Eric said to me, "We've been called to that same apartment several times before. Last spring there was a guy who used to jump out the third-story apartment onto the sidewalk. One day, he finally 'bought the farm' [died] though."

Later in the day I asked Eric why he had thought that the run to the apartment house was going to be a crock run.

Eric: Well there were three things in my way of thinking. First,

I recognized the address of the apartment. That's where the guy used to jump out the window. Then, the code [drug overdose] didn't fit with the fire department being called, too. And the call from the box for a fire truck was suspicious. It all added up to a crock!

Researcher: Does that kind of thing bother you?

Eric: A little—but you get used to it. You're going to get some of those once in a while.

Another problem with the crock run is that sometimes these patients ask to be taken to an emergency room, and the EMTs must transport someone who is not an emergency case and risk the displeasure of the emergency-room nurses who must find temporarily a place for someone they feel is not a legitimate case. Paramedics rarely transport a crock since they are concerned only with life-threatened cases. If a patient does not warrant their attention, they can turn the case over to the district EMTs for transportation.

The following vignette points to the problem of transporting nonsick patients to a hospital emergency room:

One morning while riding with a district EMT ambulance crew, we had a run to a gas station, not far from County Hospital. A black service-station attendant had called the ambulance. We arrived and found a woman, who looked to be middle-aged, heavyset, sitting behind the wheel of a late-model car. She was crying, and told Harry and Art—the EMTs—that she felt sick.

Woman: I've just been to the emergency room at Mercy, because my ankles were hurting and they said I was well enough to go home. But I got sick again, and pulled in here [the service station].

Art checked her vital signs and asked her several questions about her health and examined her ankles. He told her that her blood pressure was a little high, but other than that she was OK.

Woman: I want you to take me to County, but I can't leave my car. Can't you drive me in my car?

Harry: We can't do that. If you want us to take you to County, you'll have to go in the ambulance.

Woman (crying): But what about my car? It's brand-new and I don't want to leave it to get stolen!

Service-Station Attendant: You can't leave it here, lady!

While all this was taking place, a Metro-City policeman arrived, and he suggested that the woman phone a relative to come and get her car, and let the ambulance take her to the hospital. When we arrived at the County Hospital emergency room, a nurse met us at the door, and Harry explained the woman's situation:

Harry: She's been to Mercy emergency room this morning for pain in her ankles, and they told her she was well enough to drive home. But she says she is too weak to drive.

The nurse glared at Harry and told the EMTs to take the woman to an examining room. It was evident that the nurse was far from happy with Harry and Art.

In the above illustration, the nurse was displeased because this woman had already been through an emergency-room examination at another hospital in Metro-City. Since the Mercy Hospital emergency room had found no medical reason to admit the woman, she became the problem of the County Hospital emergency room. The nurse was visibly upset with Harry and Art because she expected them to handle such a case in the street and avoid having the patient admitted to her jurisdiction. Art and Harry for their part knew they were bringing a crock to the County emergency room, but since the patient insisted on going, they had little choice.

HOUSE CALLS

Another category of runs that EMTs and paramedics make and that they consider inappropriate are what one paramedic referred to as house calls. These runs are for victims of very minor cuts and bruises or other complaints that many persons would take to a doctor's office, or in by-gone years would have been treated by a doctor at the patient's home. Most of the people who call for emergency ambulance service are usually too poor, too uninformed, or too physically incapacitated to take advantage of the medical-care system designed for general, nonacute medical problems. For such people, there is no private family doctor to turn to; they cannot afford one. For them and for others who are bedridden, alone, and frightened, an emergency ambulance crew is the only source of medical attention possible.

The latter group—the elderly, the shut-ins, the physically disabled—constitutes an interesting type of emergency patient. Metro-City (and many other cities of its size) has many people living within its borders who are alone, poor, chronically ill, and often frightened about the state of their health. They are found in cheap run-down apartments, dilapidated rooming houses, and skid-row hotels. When they need medical attention and/or become anxious about their health, they often call an ambulance, or others in the building, who care enough, call for them. Usually what such persons need is general medical attention, but they are unable to get to a satisfactory medical source. Someone must come to them, and this is often an EMT or paramedic crew. Such persons have learned that when they feel badly or in some other way need attention, an emergency ambulance will respond. The phone call always works; someone will always come to examine the patient. The patient will have someone to talk to about his or her health, his or her aches and pains, and if he or she wants the comfort of being in a hospital for a while, he or she can ask to be transported to an emergency room. In this sense, the emergency ambulance system allows some people access to the health-care system who otherwise would be unable to get into it.

An elderly skid row alcoholic who wants to go to a hospital to dry out, a bedridden and neglected man with angina pain who wants his fears allayed that he is not dying, an elderly woman who cannot seem to keep warm and thinks she is sick—these are the kinds of house calls that EMT ambulance crews make. Some of the patients will be transported at their request; others will receive an examination and their medical history will be briefly recorded. But all will get some kind of attention—and for many that is all they wanted anyway.

The following two vignettes taken from my field notes may serve as an illustration of the house call.

This afternoon while riding with Alan and Bill, two EMTs working a district ambulance, the dispatcher gave us a run for a "sick person." We went to an apartment in the inner city near the downtown area. The apartment building had plastic sheets taped over the windows in place of storm windows. We climbed wooden, uncarpeted stairs to the second floor where several black people were standing, two of them with their arms around a middle-aged-looking black male who was shaking.

Alan asked the people if there was somewhere we could sit down so they could examine the man. One of the men opened the door to an apartment and said it was his place. We walked into the apartment and everyone followed (about six people). The man who was shaking sat on the couch. There were three rooms—a bedroom, a kitchen, and living room. The walls were bare and unpainted with plaster chipping. The floors were uncarpeted and strewn with cigarette butts, soft-drink cans, and papers. The furniture in the living room was broken with springs sticking out of the chairs and the couch. Alan and Bill asked the patient questions about his health, but all the man would say was that he was forty-two years old. An older woman who said she was his lady friend, said they found him lying in the snow in some sort of seizure.

Woman: You know he's usually drunk, and when he's not drinking, he gets real nervous. He was nervous today, and that probably is why he fell in the snow.

After some minutes of examination, Alan suggested that the patient see a doctor. The man said finally that he wouldn't go to a hospital. Alan asked the woman if she had a car and could take him to a clinic. She said she didn't have one, but she would do what she could. Bill asked the patient to sign a release form, which he did, and after telling the patient to see a doctor, we left.

The second example of the house call occurred during a paramedic ambulance run for a patient with a possible heart attack.

I was riding as an observer with Tony and Linda, two paramedics who had worked as partners for some time. The address turned out to be a walk-up apartment building; a woman met us at the entrance, and we went up to the second floor. The woman said she was the manager of the building, and that she had called the ambulance at the request of one of the tenants.

We entered an apartment that was small, cluttered, and very warm. The living room contained a large double bed where an elderly man lay in his pajamas. He looked tired, pale, and anxious. He said that earlier in the morning he experienced pain in the left arm and had taken a nitroglycerin tablet and was now feeling better. He said he was worried, so he had the manager call an ambulance.

Tony and Linda attached the heart monitor to the man for an EKG reading and took his vital signs. Tony asked the patient many questions about his pain, his general health, and how he felt. He suggested that the man agree to go with them to the hospital for a checkup, but the man said he felt better and would call them again if he needed help. As we were leaving, Linda took the apartment manager aside and told her to check on the man from time to time.

I asked Linda if the patient was sick.

"He's not really that sick," she said, "but he wanted some company and attention. He's such a nice old man—so you give it to him."

As you can see from the above examples, while housecalls are considered inappropriate by EMTs and paramedics since they do not constitute bona fide medical emergencies, the EMTs and paramedics at County expected to get a certain amount of these runs. They came to realize that without their attention these people would be truly alone and abandoned. There is also always the chance that some house calls can become appropriate runs. If the ambulance crew that responds feels that the patient needs to see a doctor they may even try to persuade the patient to let them transport him or her. Note that in the second example cited above, Tony wanted to transport the patient. If the patient had agreed, the status of the run would have been elevated to an appropriate run, since it would have been a transport case, one that was urged by the paramedic crew.

TAXI SERVICE

The third category of inappropriate runs concerns only the EMT crews in district ambulances. The EMTs at County Hospital pointed out on several occasions that many persons in Metro-City used the ambulance service as a way of getting to their clinic appointments at County Hospital. As in the second category described above, these persons are usually the poor, the disabled, and the elderly who often do not have any other means of transportation to get themselves to the hospital. They have learned to use the emergency-care system to their advantage by having a friend or relative call for an emergency ambulance and report a "sick person." When EMTs receive a Code 6 from the dispatcher, experience has shown them that Code 6 can be almost any type of sick person. It might be someone critically ill, requiring paramedic attention, or it might be the exact opposite—someone who feels sick shortly before he or she is due to keep a hospital appointment. There is little that EMT crews can do about such runs, for often these patients have a chronic illness and therefore require some medical attention; and since they request transportation, this cannot be refused by the EMTs.

Earlier in this chapter, an EMT at County Hospital who was acting as driver for a paramedic unit, rather than work on a district ambulance, said that she preferred the former duty to the latter, because of "all the bullshit you see in the districts." In part, the taxi-service function is one of the aspects that she was referring to.

We have looked rather closely at those types of runs that are considered inappropriate, but that must be contended with as part of emergency ambulance work; there remains a final category of runs that are thought to be legitimate demands for emergency care, but which because of several related circumstances, produce a sense of futility among the EMTs and paramedics. These runs provide opportunities for skill utilization, but the physical condition of the patient is already so deteriorated that there is little hope for a save, or any kind of success-ful outcome. In part they are emergency exercises in futility, and I therefore refer to this category of events as futile runs.

FUTILE RUNS

Paramedics, like those who trained at and worked for County Hospi-tal, have many techniques and much equipment at their disposal, which they use to help those who are critically ill or injured. Earlier we saw the importance of the save in the paramedic scheme of values—those occasions calling for heroic medical efforts through which the life of a patient is restored. The elation of the save is always balanced, however, by the disappointment and futility of the misses and near misses—those occasions when an all-out effort is expended on a patient whose medical condition is so hopeless that the paramedics have little or no chance for success.

I have chosen three examples of futile runs to illustrate slightly differ-ent conditions and situations but in all of which, by and large, the emergency ambulance crew had the odds stacked against them. Para-medics, as we have seen, try to create advantages for themselves whenever they can in performing their work so that it will be successful. In the following runs, no advantage could be created by the paramedics in-volved, in a sense they had little control over the events surrounding the run, and this lack of control contributed to the sense of futility. The first example concerns a run for a cardiac-arrest victim, which always has the potential for a save, but on this run, a series of circumstances put the paramedics at what they considered a decided disadvantage:

> During the evening shift on a paramedic unit, the dispatcher gave the crew a run to assist a nearby township volunteer-ambulance unit on a cardiac-arrest victim. This is a fairly common occurrence, and Andy, the driver, sped through the city streets at high speed, since he admitted it would take us a while to get there. We found the address in the township, a small frame bungalow, with several emergency vehicles parked in front. We entered the living room and found a middle-aged man lying on the floor, and a young woman (township EMT volunteer) was performing chest massage on the man, while a young male volunteer forced air into the man's lungs with a bagmask.

> Alan and Vic, the County paramedics, began to unload their equipment while the volunteers from the township told them about the patient's condition. Alan attached the heart monitor

and prepared to defibrillate the patient to induce a normal heart rhythm. Vic laid out endotracheal instruments and began to intubate the patient which took a few minutes. The defibrillation was attempted by Alan several times, but no normal rhythm was obtained. Alan said, "We better go in with him," and asked the patient's wife what hospital she preferred. The patient was loaded into the paramedic ambulance, and Alan told the woman volunteer from the township to continue her compressions. Alan drove the ambulance into County "signal ten" [red lights and siren] since there were three paramedics on duty on the crew that night and two stayed in the rear to monitor the patient. En route to the hospital, Alan turned to me:

Alan: You know Jim, years ago people just passed away. But now they have cardiac arrests, and we go out and beat on them—but the result is usually pretty much the same.

Researcher: There won't be any save on this one?

Alan: Well the problem is that the guy has been "down" too long. That township uses volunteers, and by the time the volunteers get to a person's house usually too much time has elapsed—if a guy's in "arrest." Then by the time we get out there, you've added another twenty minutes or so. We'll take him into Mercy, but they won't work on him too long. We try the electroshock to get a regular heart rhythm, but if we can't get a normal rhythm the first two or three times, there's not much hope.

In the above case, the paramedics involved badly wanted to achieve a save, but the case was complicated by several factors. First of all, since they had to travel to the township, their response time was slow, and for a cardiac-arrest run, this is a decided disadvantage. Second, the patient's family lived in a volunteer ambulance community, and it takes longer for a volunteer ambulance to reach a patient as first responders. Alan became aware that the odds were not in favor of achieving a save and thus became rather philosophical with me en route to the hospital. His sense of futility can be seen in his statement, "The result is pretty much the same," forgetting temporarily the saves he had participated in during the course of his career.

The second example focuses on the problem of emergency runs for patients dying of chronic, terminal disease for whom successful resuscitation means only a brief postponement of the inevitable:

During the second shift, I was riding as an observer with the supervisor, a paramedic by the name of Phillip. We took a run from the dispatcher for a "sick person," and found the address at a small house on the east side of Metro-City. The patient was an elderly man, lying in bed, receiving oxygen from a unit mounted in the bedroom. We were joined at the scene by a district ambulance crew. The patient was very pale, thin, and emaciated-looking. After Phillip examined the patient, he started an IV in the man's arm, and we transported the patient to a nearby veteran's hospital. Later in the evening, I asked Phillip about the patient.

Researcher: Do you think he'll live?

Phillip: There's an interesting run. We knew the patient was dying. His wife told me that he was a terminal cancer patient for years. They brought him home so he wouldn't die in the hospital. Here is a case where we're damned if we do—and damned if we don't. The patient is waiting to die—this is what he is supposed to do. But at the moment, someone calls the "wonder boys" with their "wonder drugs" to resuscitate the patient. So we revive him—so he can have a few more weeks of pain. We get a lot of calls like that. Sometimes the family doesn't tell us the patient is terminal, until we've spent half the night trying to revive someone!

In the above illustration, the temporal dimension provides an interesting contrast to the first example. In the first case, when the ambulance crew arrived too late to make a save, the time perspective was measured in minutes. In the second example, the paramedics were also too late but as measured in terms of weeks and months; here the patient is in the final stages of a dying trajectory that would take a long period of time to accomplish, and there was little that the County paramedics and EMTs could do beyond a temporary revival and postponement of death.

The third example focuses on those runs that start out as successful, certain, and predictable but end up in unforseeable tragedy, despite the paramedic team's best efforts:

The following conversation took place one afternoon in dispatch communications at County Hospital.

Vic (a paramedic, talking to the EMT dispatcher): We had a run last night, picked up a thirty-five-year-old female patient who almost drowned in a tub of hot water. I guess she had taken some drug, antidepressant or something, and climbed into the tub. It was given out as a district run, but when they got there, they sent for the medic. When we got to her, I thought sure she was going to make it, and all I did was monitor to the hospital. Everything was going smooth until we got right outside St. Regis, and she "arrested." I mean she just went right out. But we get her back before we took her into the ER.

Dispatcher: Is she going to make it?

Vic: It depends on what you mean by making it. She's on a respirator.

Here Vic displays his dismay at a case that looked successful and routine but one that without warning ended in tragedy. Although Vic and his crew were able to resuscitate the young woman and restore a heartbeat, the patient who was on a respirator was in critical condition. For Vic there were two futile dimensions involved in this run: one, the resuscitation was only partially successful for the patient was now in a coma; and, two, a patient who was expected to recover and who Vic thought "was going to make it" suddenly "arrested" only seconds away from the door of the emergency facility. In such a run, little reward or satisfaction can be gained by Vic and his crew. A matter of seconds and minutes was all that stood between success and futility, and here this crew shares the fate of Alan and his partners in our first example. However, Alan had a nagging suspicion, as we sped swiftly through the streets of Metro-City and he counted the minutes tick off en route, that we might be too late to get a save. He knew, and admitted later, that time was not on the ambulance crew's side. Vic and his crew were also the victims of time, though of another sort. Without knowing it, their patient too had little time left. But in a deceptive way, the patient's signs were good, and all pointed to a routine transport to St. Regis Hospital. Then within seconds and without warning, a successful run was lost and attempts to save the patient were futile. This is what it means to do emergency ambulance work, to tread constantly the thin line between success and failure.

Having examined in some detail, the various ways in which emergency ambulance runs are evaluated and given meaning by the EMTs and paramedics at County Hospital, it is now appropriate to look at some of the wider and more general values. These more general values focus not only on runs but also on those aspects of emergency ambulance work through which meaning and value are directed. It is time to explore further how EMTs and paramedics view their work, their patients, and themselves.

SPECIAL PATIENTS

For many years now we have known that emergency health-care workers make moral and social judgments about the worth of their patients.[12] Not all patients are treated alike; some are considered more worthy of medical services than others. These judgments about the social and moral worth of patients are sometimes made on the basis of the socioeconomic status of the patient, their community "importance," racial characteristics, and such demographic considerations as age and sex. Much of the research literature demonstrates that health-care workers see those patients who are young, middle-class, important, and white as more worthy of care and sympathy. Such patients receive more prompt attention, more considerate service, and in some circumstances, even more heroic emergency medical care.

The paramedics and EMTs who worked for County Hospital also made judgments about the value of those people they were called upon to help. Their categories of worthiness were, however, not very clearly defined or extensive. Socioeconomic status, sex, and community importance did not seem to be major considerations in the amount of effort spent to save an emergency victim. Nor did race seem to be an important factor. The major variable about patient status appeared to be age, and when defining someone as a special patient, age was the ascendant element.

County EMTs and paramedics held children to be worthy of their finest efforts. Emergency runs involving children were nearly always considered important, and many special efforts were made to insure the health and safety of child patients. Youthful victims of disease and injury evoked not only a sympathetic response, but also a careful attention to medical detail, concern with the emotional state and fears of the victim, and if the case required, all-out medical efforts. The treatment of children as special people by ambulance workers can be seen by looking at three dimensions involved in their care; directing sympathy toward the victim; attempting to alleviate a patient's fears and apprehensions; and making a medical judgment about resuscitation efforts.

In an earlier chapter I described how paramedics and EMTs learn to suppress their emotions and block out their feelings toward victims of medical emergencies. EMTs and paramedics become hardened in their work, so that their sympathy and feelings toward the suffering of patients do not interfere with their ability to deliver cool and speedy medical care. Child victims of accidents, illness, abuse, and neglect, however, often evoke feelings of sympathy and concern on the part of ambulance personnel. Ethan, an EMT who had worked for County for about a year, expressed his attitudes toward children in this way:

> I really get bothered when children get hurt, because I've got two daughters of my own. I think about them when I see children get hurt. Whenever I hear the dispatcher say, "Medic II, District II—child injured," I get apprehensive. On the way to the scene, I wonder what it will be. I always hope it won't be too bad.

In their work paramedics and EMTs confront many child victims of abuse, neglect, and outright abandonment who evoke a strongly sympathetic response from them; coping with these feelings is often very difficult for them. Very often, too, there is little that can be done for such victims, and that further frustrates their efforts since they feel strongly about a patient whom they cannot even help. Vince, an experienced paramedic, talked to me about his past experiences and his emotional response:

> In the last two years I've seen four dead children, victims of child abuse. You remember those. Those you keep track of. You really feel bad—especially when you know someone killed them. Older people, it's not so bad when they get it—you figure they've lived a full life. And the attitudes of parents really bother me too.
>
> We had a run last year, two children had overdosed without their mother knowing it. When we got there, one child had been dead so long we didn't even start. As we worked on the other, the mother sat on the couch smoking like there was nothing going on! We were able to resuscitate, but the kid was in a coma for months. That night after the mother had been charged for child neglect, in front of the TV cameras, she started crying, "My babies." What a hypocrite!

This kind of attitude on the part of EMTs and paramedics often gets translated into special forms of occupational behavior in which efforts are expended on behalf of a child that would not occur if the patient were an older person. Paramedics and EMTs call this "going out of their way" to be of help, and it involves special exertions which bring few rewards to the ambulance crew but are expended anyway because the child victim is considered special. Sid, a district-ambulance EMT described such an occasion:

> We had a run yesterday that was interesting. We were dispatched to a house where a six-year-old boy had cut his foot on some glass. It had stopped bleeding by the time we got there. The baby sitter appeared to be dumb, and didn't seem to know what was going on. The mother was out of town and couldn't be reached, and the father was at work and no one knew how to get in touch with him. Someone at the house mentioned the boy had a heart murmur, and with the cut on the foot, I got worried about infection. The baby sitter said the last time the boy cut himself he was in the hospital for weeks.
>
> I wasn't sure what to do. The house was filthy—garbage all over the floors with broken glass. I called the Youth Hospital and explained the situation to a doctor there, and she said to bring him in. Then I called the dispatcher and told him about my problem, and he put us out of service.

It turned out to be a mess. The baby sitter didn't know any-thing—I couldn't find anyone legally responsible to sign papers to take the child to the hospital. So I packed them all up and took them to the hospital. It was a real pain, but I just couldn't leave the kid in that house till a doctor looked at him. The dispatcher wasn't too pleased.

Sid—and he is not unique in his attitude—had another occasion to show how his concern for children influenced his decisions to make special efforts he would not otherwise make. The following serves as an illustration:

I was riding on a paramedic unit when the dispatcher told us to assist a district at a city location. We arrived at the scene, a grocery store parking lot, and a district unit was parked there with red lights on and motor running. We entered the district ambulance, and a teen-age girl lay on the cot, and the EMTs described for the paramedics the condition of the patient. I asked Sid, one of the district EMTs on duty, what was involved.

Sid: She was shopping in the store and started to get chest pain and hyperventilation. We examined her and everything looks OK, and she is feeling better now—but I don't want to take a chance with kids. I've got a soft spot with them. I'll give kids every chance. That's why I called for a medic unit, so they could run an EKG, and make sure about things.

In the above example, Sid was placing himself in a potentially difficult position. Normally, district ambulance units request paramedic assistance only when they are fairly certain a patient needs advanced life support. Sid was not sure if the paramedics were needed, but what influenced his decision was the patient's age. In short, Sid's judgment was based on the idea that when the patient is young and when in doubt, call for a paramedic unit. As it turned out, the paramedics decided to transport the girl to Youth Hospital, and they transferred the patient in the paramedic ambulance. What happened on the way to the hospital demonstrates the second feature of children as special patients, and concerns those attempts to alleviate the fears and anxieties of young patients—efforts that are not normally carried out to such an extent on behalf of adult patients.

The following sequence is taken from my field notes and describes what transpired as the paramedic transported the young victim referred to above:

The paramedics on duty—George and Dale—decided that they should take the girl to Youth Hospital for an examination. They put her into the medic unit, and we proceeded in. I rode in the rear compartment with George and the patient, who was connected to the heart monitor. George engaged the girl in conversation; he quietly joked and kidded with her about her school activities, her home life, and her boyfriends.

George: Sue, look at that scope there. That shows your heartbeat. You see you're normal. Isn't that something? This guy sitting back here is Jim. Sue meet Jim. He is our sociologist; he observes us. Have you ever met a sociologist before?

The patient answered George's questions quietly and soon asked a few of her own. Later, after we had checked her into the emergency room, and were en route back to County Hospital, George told me, "I talk to kids like that because it seems to make them feel better. It gets her mind off her pain and calms her down. I didn't want her hyperventilating."

Such quiet and relaxed behavior on George's part was a bit unusual as observation had shown that he was normally a direct, no-nonsense type of paramedic. He was not given to a great deal of conversation with patients that was not directly related to their health or medical problems. With youthful victims, however, his attitude tended to soften.

The final way in which young people evoke special response from EMTs and paramedics concern decisions about resuscitation efforts. Since age appears to be a crucial factor, I have included the discussion in this section, but because the problem of medical heroics has a broader dimension to it, I will discuss it under the heading Tough Decisions.

TOUGH DECISIONS

Paramedics are generally the first responders to life-threatening medical emergencies, and it is among their responsibilities to provide advanced life support. Many of the patients they find at the emergency scene are near death, without pulse or heartbeat. Paramedics must begin immediate resuscitation measures if the patient is to be revived, and such measures, as we have already seen, are not always successful. Paramedics argue that some of their greatest rewards accompany a save or resuscitation. Conversely, as noted earlier, unsuccessful attempts can bring about a sense of futility.

The paramedics at County Hospital tried to create advantages for themselves in resuscitation efforts, realizing that not all such attempts will be successful and that some patients stand a better chance of being revived than others. Conversations with experienced paramedics and my own field observations reveal that decisions regarding whether or not to start resuscitation procedures at the scene were considered problematic. However, such decisions must be made, and three criteria appear to form the basis of these decisions: the age of the victim; assumptions about the nature of disease processes; and the consequences for the patient.

The age of the victim is considered important, since as we have already seen, it is assumed that younger victims are better able to withstand the rigors of resuscitation, and because of their youth, have a brighter future. In addition, the nature of the disease process is thought to be important since if a person is in the final stages of a degenerative disease process, it is unlikely resuscitation will be successful. Because older persons are more prone to degenerative diseases, they are considered "less viable" for resuscitation. And finally, if paramedics think that the consequences of a successful resuscitation are less desirable than death, a victim is "better off" dead. For example, if paramedics feel that a victim has little chance for a full recovery then resuscitation efforts might not be in the best interests of the patient. These ideas are clearly demonstrated in a conversation conducted with Eric, a seasoned County Hospital paramedic, who discussed his feelings regarding resuscitation attempts:

Researcher: Will you start resuscitation efforts on all victims?

Eric: Actually we'll give a kid more leeway than an older person. They still have a relatively long life in front of them. If they're [the victims] eighty or ninety, they've lived their life. If we give them a year or two, it's not going to help them that much. Their age is against them too, If they have had a major disease that caused the death, it's a natural death. Kids usually don't die from natural causes; they die from accidents.

Researcher: How else is the idea of death involved?

Eric: Death is just the end stage of living. So many EMTs see death as "My God, this isn't to be allowed in our world. We can't have this; we have to save everybody!" Well, some people with long-standing illnesses have no hope even if you resuscitate them. They'll just suffer. Because they not only have the problem they had before, but you've compounded it with fractured ribs and lack of oxygen to the brain. Better sometimes to just let them go. Sad, but true.

Researcher: When does a person have their age working against them?

Eric: We divide it into young people and old people. Old people in our criteria are anyone in their late sixties and up.

Researcher: Do all paramedics follow this?

Eric: Well, partly it's a problem of street experience. Some of the younger guys will resuscitate anybody at the drop of a hat. If you know that if you can get the guy or girl back but they are just going to be a vegetable, why bother? A big medical expense for the family, years of grief—it's a hell of a decision to have to make, I'll tell you. Someone has to make it, and we're stuck with it.

CONCLUSION

This chapter has been concerned with the inside world of the ambulance-riding EMT and paramedic, how they see their work, their patients, and themselves. In a sense it has been a description of their joys and rewards, tribulations, failures, and futilities.

We must remember that only fifteen years ago there were no EMTs and paramedics. Ambulance runs were mostly a matter of transportation and basic first aid, racing against time to get an emergency victim to the hospital. The whole philosophy of emergency medical service has since changed. Through the role and the work of EMTs and paramedics, at least part of hospital-based emergency medical care can now be administered at the emergency scene, if the patient cannot be taken to the hospital quickly enough. Thus the emergence of the new medical role of EMT and paramedic, who at an ever-increasing rate are learning to bring the latest in emergency medical care to the emergency victim.

It appears, however, that once the older traditional model of getting a patient and swiftly running him or her to the hospital was abandoned, what emerged was a group of men and women with sufficient medical training to "do something" for the patient while at the scene and on the way to the hospital. The patient is still transported, but he or she is also now being given life-support emergency medical care. Those who peform the work, having some degree of training and commitment, have begun to acquire many of the values and attitudes found in other medical workers. Emergency victims are referred to as patients, desires to put acquired skills and techniques into practice become increasingly important, and expectations about being of real medical help to patients begin to escalate. EMTs and paramedics begin to evaluate cases on the same basis that doctors and nurses do: To what degree does this case fit my conception of my proper role and obligation? Perhaps this is the first step in achieving a firm occupational identity. At any rate few EMTs and paramedics now seem content to provide transportation only. They have developed a strong service ideology in which their need to be of medical help to others forms a large part of the occupational ethos.

Yet, as we have seen, the element of uncertainty looms large in their work along with the certainty of risk and danger. On the one hand, EMTs and paramedics can be sure that the risks and dangers associated with their work will never really diminish; those who work in the street learn to accept this. On the other hand, to the degree that emergency ambulance crews and those they work for expect them to do something medically valuable for patients, they must face the uncertainties inherent in medical practice. If uncertainty is a significant problem for physicians, it must also be one for paramedics.

One final note in closing: In the past several years there has been a marked tendency for health-care workers to specialize. We have seen this especially in nursing and among physicians. The doctor, for example, is no longer "all things to all patients." He or she now limits his or her practice as a way of reducing uncertainty, and this also has eliminated many of the problems of the generalist.

The EMTs and paramedics working for County Hospital want to specialize in emergency medicine. As we have seen, they want to bring their skills and abilities to help people in what they consider to be legitimate medical emergencies. Yet there is a latent or secondary dimension to their work, and that is bringing into the health-care system those who otherwise would not get there, giving care and attention to the neglected and forgotten. It has been said that social workers are in part responsible for "patching up" socially and psychologically those who have been brutalized by the socioeconomic system, especially the poor. The counterpart of the social worker in the field of health-care seems to be the urban EMT and paramedic. When the EMT and paramedic bring medical attention to the so-called crock, administer to abused and neglected children, and make house calls on the elderly and urban poor, they are patching up the failures of modern health-care systems— and, I suppose, in an even larger sense they daily witness the failures of modern society.

The paramedic or EMT brings to the bedside of an elderly man some of the best of what contemporary emergency medicine has to offer— e.g., electronic heart monitors and drugs. Yet, in getting to the patient's bedside, as they climb two flights of dilapidated stairs, brush by the urinal pots in a building with no plumbing, notice that there are no sheets on the patient's bed in an apartment barely fit for human habitation, can these paramedics not help but become aware of the irony of their work: that in making this house call they are bringing only a small part of what this patient really needs to fulfill his life, that we live in a society that invests more in heart monitors than in the lives of people who need enrichment in so many ways? But the paramedics and EMTs at County made and continue to make the run, to rush to the bedside and give human contact and response to someone desperately in need. And while these EMTs and paramedics may not recognize it, since it is not "real emergency medicine," for many persons in the backrooms of Metro-City this may well be their most rewarding service.

6

PROFESSIONALISM AND THE
EMT AND PARAMEDIC

In an earlier chapter, we stated that some of the values that permeate the work of the EMT and paramedic are professional. Does this mean that emergency ambulance work is an emerging profession? If so, just what is meant when sociologists talk about a profession?

It is not easy to define exactly what a profession is. In part it can be considered a label that sets some occupations apart from others. It also has to do with the idea of esteem or prestige that the community gives to certain occupations. In a sense, a professional occupation has successfully created an image of itself as having a high degree of esteem and prestige. In discussions of professions, however, there is also the notion that a true profession performs some public service that requires specialized knowledge and skill; thus those who are part of a given profession are able to exert a powerful control over how that service will be performed. A professional occupation then exists partly through public need and acceptance of some needed service and partly through its own pervasive authority to determine the shape and content of that service.

Those who study health-care workers are aware that one of the prevailing models used to understand occupational behavior is that of being a professional. Perhaps this is because the field of health care is dominated by one of the most successful and powerful professionals in the world—that of medicine. Emerging health-care workers, as a result, see their opportunities for acceptance, power, and financial success as contingent upon the degree to which they are able to professionalize. In this sense, emergency medical ambulance crews are no exception among health-care workers.

Several scholars in sociology have attempted to describe and define the essential elements of a profession, or those characteristics differentiating one occupation apart from another.[13] Some have emphasized the idea of service orientation and abstract knowledge; others have argued the importance of licensure and of a code of ethics; still others have suggested that those in a profession occupy a dominant position in the division of labor, insuring control over the shape of work. Each of these theses has its supporters and detractors, and each seems to have some measure of empirical validity and predictive value in understanding occupational behavior. In analyzing the potential for professional development of the contemporary EMT and paramedic, I would like to draw upon them and suggest that the following variables are particularly important; prolonged training and education; development of specialized skills; a collective orientation; licensure and a code of ethics.

My argument is that occupations characterized by these features are thought to be more professional than those occupations that lack them. Professions can become powerful forces in society, in shaping how work in certain areas will be performed. This seems to be especially true of medicine and the law. Since the profession of medicine is said to owe much of its success, power, and prestige to its ability to be the preeminent profession, those occupations in the field of health care that want such rewards, try to emulate the professional model. To be an EMT or paramedic is among the newest occupations in the field of medicine, and an important question becomes, To what degree is it an emerging or "budding" profession? Will its future success and acceptance in medicine rise and fall on its ability to take on professional characteristics? In the section that follows, I will examine those aspects of the work and role of the EMTs and paramedics at County that have a bearing on their capability to professionalize. I will suggest that EMTs and paramedics have some rudimentary professional features, yet the pressures toward unionization tend to complicate the picture. I will begin by looking at the elements of the professional process as they apply.

PROLONGED TRAINING AND EDUCATION

The amount of training and education needed to become certified as an EMT or paramedic is certainly less than that required in the more established licensed professions, such as the law, medicine, nursing, or teaching. Moreover, the EMT and paramedic training requirements vary from state to state, despite national efforts for standardization. As we have seen the EMTs at County must have some 81 to 150 hours of basic instruction; the paramedics, nearly 800 hours of advanced instruction.

It is doubtful that education of this limited duration will result in the deeply internalized professional values and commitments that one finds in the law, for example, with its three years of postgraduate education. Also, as most EMT and paramedics at County argued, their training prepared them only in the most basic way for what they confront in the streets; much of what they come to know about their work is acquired through direct experience rather than through formal education. In light of this, one EMT-paramedic instructor at County Hospital argued that EMTs and paramedics should be the ones to control their instruction rather than doctors and nurses.

> *Ethan:* I feel that EMT and paramedic instruction should come from EMTs and paramedics who have had experience in the streets. And I think this is now beginning to happen because we know that on-the-street medicine is entirely different from in-house medicine.

For EMTs and paramedics, education does not end with completion of the advanced life-support instruction. County Hospital, for example, requires every paramedic to complete thirteen hours of in-service training per month for their yearly certification. Some paramedics welcome this additional opportunity for training; others feel it is an additional burden. Those with a fairly strong professional orientation feel that the in-service training is necessary to emulate the more successful medical professions.

Alan, an experienced paramedic and part-time supervisor at County Hospital expressed his eagerness for in-service training:

> I feel that our thirteen-hour-a-month required in-service is fine. Hell, if doctors have to do it, why shouldn't we? Things are changing so fast in our field, how else are we going to keep up? One month they tell us one way to do something, and the next month it's something else. We need that training.

Although the basic education is attenuated, the philosophy behind in-service training connotes a concern with professionalism. Yet because most of what is really considered important to know is learned on the job, the role of education in promoting professional commitments for EMTs and paramedics is limited.

SKILLS AND TECHNIQUES

One of the features that is thought to distinguish a profession is the degree of esoteric skill required. In other words, does an occupation involve knowledge and application of skills that are highly sophisticated and not shared by the general public? Professional work is technical, in the sense that lay people are ignorant of those particular specialized skills and dependent upon the professional to apply these highly valued techniques and procedures.

In their training and in their work, EMTs and paramedics acquire skills and techniques that are not shared by the general public. While there is much talk today about laymen learning cardiopulmonary resuscitation skills, most of the public is ignorant of this basic technique.

The nature of emergency medical training is such that EMTs and paramedics learn fairly sophisticated skills in patient care, but because of their limited education, the theoretical knowledge behind those skills is usually not provided. EMTs and paramedics working for County, for example, are taught certain techniques that only a few short years ago would have been performed exclusively by physicians. Today EMTs and paramedics perform them as part of their daily routine without six years of medical training. Without going into all the reasons for this transformation, it seems apparent that such techniques—inserting endotracheal tubes, starting IVs, administering drugs, taking electrocardiographs—can be learned and performed successfully without understanding or knowing their theoretical medical foundations. While the medical knowledge of the EMT and paramedic is not extensive and esoteric, the techniques learned are sophisticated enough often to obtain quite dramatic results.

COLLECTIVITY ORIENTATION

Probably the strongest aspect of professionalism voiced among the emergency ambulance workers at County Hospital was their concern for "good patient care," which meant putting the needs of the patient ahead of their own. One of the hallmarks of being a professional is this willingness to devote oneself to the needs of the client and to subordinate one's own self-interests. The assumption is that the client requires the services of the professional because lacking specialized skills and knowledge they cannot help themselves; the professional, in turn, does not take advantage of this situation, but acts on behalf and in the best interests of whoever seeks help. Also involved is the idea that the professional should serve all in the community who need his or her services and be blind to distinctions of class, color, sex, or ethnicity. County EMTs and paramedics indicated repeatedly that the most rewarding aspect of their work lay in helping people.

It is not clearly evident just where this orientation among EMTs and paramedics comes from—whether it is inculcated during training, whether those with a strong service orientation are self-selecting; or whether it is learned on the job. But among the majority of EMTs and paramedics observed and interviewed, it was present.

The idea of good patient care gets expressed in many ways in the daily routines of EMTs and paramedics from all-out heroic medical efforts to save a life to the soothing, comforting words spoken to a young child or elderly woman frightened by illness or injury. It is also reflected in the way that EMTs and paramedics evaluate emergency hospital rooms, whether the emergency-room doctors and nurses are thought to be "aggressive" in their care of the patients that the ambulance workers bring in. For example, if a patient is brought in who has cardiac arrest, and the paramedics have worked on the patient all the way from the scene to their arrival at the hospital, they expect the emergency-room doctors also to continue all-out efforts. If the doctors give up after an initial unsuccessful attempt at resuscitation, the paramedics feel that the emergency-room staff is not as committed to patient care as it should be. Possibly on future runs that particular emergency facility will be avoided in a case of cardiac arrest.

Another demonstration of collective orientation is evident in the fact that EMTs and paramedics rarely if ever complain of the uncomfortable, unappealing, if not appalling conditions under which they must occasionally work. Heat, cold, dangerous risks, are all adapted to and accepted if a patient is judged in need of emergency medical care. EMTs and paramedics are rarely concerned with their own comfort and safety if the patient has a legitimate need for their services. No run is ever refused, no patient is abandoned nor neglected, if the event is defined as an appropriate medical emergency. Here is a personal illustration:

I was riding with George and Vince, one of the paramedic crews; we had just transported a trauma patient to Mercy Hospital when the dispatcher gave the crew a Code 12 [gunshot]. We drove to the near northside of Metro-City and found a large crowd of people at the scene. There were several police cars, fire trucks, and television camera crews already there.

I went with the crew into a small house which was crowded with other emergency workers. An elderly black man had been shot in a hold-up attempt. George and Vince put shock pants on the patient [to help elevate the blood pressure] and carried him out to the ambulance to transport to Mercy. Vince yelled to Alan, the EMT driver, "Go easy."

On the way to Mercy one of the valve seals on the shock pants came off, and Vince said to George, "Shit, there goes his pressure!" Vince continued to swear as he and George attempted to devise a way to keep the shock pants inflated. George looked up and saw that the IV lines putting fluids into the patient's arms were getting in the patient's face; when he saw this, he told me, "Jim, keep those lines out of his face and let me know when those bags run low!"

George and Vince finally got the pants inflated again and appeared greatly relieved. At one point earlier, Vince had put his mouth over the open valve to keep air from leaking while George was fixing the valve seal. Both Vince and George worked very hard to keep the man stabilized, and the fact that the patient was an elderly black man seemed to have no bearing on their efforts to do all they could for him.

CODE OF ETHICS

Most established professions have a code of ethics that defines the moral duties and obligations of the professional toward the client. Occupations attempting to gain professional status often create a set of ethical standards as a way of persuading future clientele that their best interests will be protected. The code of ethics normally delimits proper client-professional relationships, aspects of confidentiality, and aspects of fair play with respect to competition. In a sense, a code of ethics attempts to set the moral tone of the profession in its relationship with the public and its internal control of occupational behavior. Quite often such ethical codes are drawn up by and have the endorsement of the profession's national association.

The National Association of Emergency Medical Technicians, which represents the professional interests of EMTs and paramedics throughout the country, has drawn up and now promotes a code of ethics. In fact the association sells copies of the code of ethics to interested EMTs and paramedics at conventions and other public gatherings. Most of the EMT and paramedic emergency ambulance workers at County Hospital at the time of this present study were, however, unaware of this code of ethics. In fact, few of them belonged to the national association. To a considerable degree therefore this code of ethics remained invisible and inconsequential to the majority of the ambulance crews at County Hospital.

Within recent months the Emergency Services Commission of the state in which this study was conducted has also devised a code of ethics for EMTs and paramedics. This code is still being refined and does not as yet have the power of statute. There are several provisos in the state code having to do with respecting the patient's right to dignity, privacy, and safety; promoting the health and well-being of the community; and upholding professional ideals and standards. Once again this code too is nonexistent as far as the EMTs and paramedics at County Hospital are concerned. Some may be vaguely aware of its existence, but few, if any, could describe its composition.

For all practical purposes, formalized, professional, and association-sanctioned codes of ethics have little bearing on the daily work of EMTs and paramedics. As we have seen, although many have a strong commitment toward what they consider "good patient care" and are concerned for the best interests of their patients, these standards are not derived from a clearly acknowledged and articulated code of ethics. While leaders in the national association doubtless realize the importance of an ethical code in establishing professional recognition, little that has been done in this area has reached the attention or interest of the working EMT or paramedic. It seems to be one feature of the professional process that as yet is not well developed.

LICENSURE

Licensure, which is normally the means by which those engaged in some particular occupation acquire and maintain exclusive jurisdiction to practice a technique or skill, is also a noted sociological feature of a profession. When the state issues a license to practice a skill or technique, it is, in a sense, giving that occupation a legal monopoly. The state guarantees exclusive jurisdiction to those qualified in a craft or occupation by making it illegal for the unlicensed to practice it.

Although EMT and paramedic groups are striving for national certification procedures, state licensing is not now a reality. Certification is not the same thing as licensing, and this is a crucial distinction in the professionalization process of EMTs and paramedics. With very few exceptions, the practice of EMTs and paramedics remains firmly under the control and regulation of the physician and not the state. Moreover, when the state through the workings of the Emergency Medical Services Commission creates new authorities and responsibilities for EMTs and paramedics, these are always placed under the general direction and supervision of a licensed medical doctor. In short, the skills and techniques of the EMTs and paramedics are not theirs exclusively to perform. These skills are for the most part medical techniques that the EMT and paramedic perform under supervision of the licensed physician, either directly in the emergency room or indirectly from standing orders. In either case, the physician is legally responsible, and therefore he or she is in authority. The EMT or paramedic is, in a sense, an extension of the emergency-room doctor; he or she can legally do no more than medical authority, i.e., the physician, will permit.

If a profession is defined in terms of its members exclusive control of certain techniques and of a license to practice it, then the EMTs and paramedics have a long way to go to gain professional status. The profession of medicine is not likely to permit the state to give another occupation control over techniques it now monopolizes. However, if one abandons this rather restrictive definition and broadens it to include advanced training, collectivity orientation, possessing a national association, and the like, then the emergency ambulance worker may well be seen as belonging to an emerging profession.

UNIONIZATION

While I was writing this study, the EMTs and paramedics employed by County Hospital were in the process of forming a union. This action was prompted by a series of often bitter disputes with the ambulance division administrators over such matters as salary, fringe benefits, and working hours. Most of the EMTs and paramedics I talked to and observed seemed to be favorable toward the union, although only a few actually sought and maintained key leadership positions. An important question that must now be considered is, What impact if any will the quest for a union have on the development of professional status among EMTs and paramedics?

When an occupational group attempts to advance the interests of its members, it has two alternatives: professionalization and unionization.[14] Professionalization seeks through prestige to gain and keep control and authority of a given occupation. Codes of ethics, collectivity orientation, and advanced education are in part aimed at gaining esteem from the larger community. When the community holds an occupation in high esteem, the state is more likely to grant it increased authority and control through such mechanisms as licensure. Unionization, on the other hand, involves collective action by an occupational group to advance its own interests and power. Strikes and the threat of the withdrawal of services are ultimate weapons in gaining the workers' demands.

Within the field of health care, doctors have gained their dominance through the process of professionalization. Nurses have also tried to promote their interests by this means, but because physicians "got there first," nurses find their own occupational authority rather restricted. Other workers, much lower in the medical hierarchy, have recently been much more likely to unionize to promote their own demands and interests. A combination of these two alternatives is, of course, a distinct possibility. In some parts of the country, nurses have sought to enhance their interests through unionization while yet retaining a strong commitment toward professionalism.

How emergency ambulance workers will promote their occupational interests remains to be seen. The occupation is of such recent development that no one can say with certainty which alternative will prevail. Unionization of community ambulance services will no doubt be used as a vehicle of power and will bring increased benefits as far as wages and working hours and conditions are concerned. In other words, when the individual ambulance worker seeks to promote his or her interests in regard to the local conditions of work, the formation of a union will be the chosen alternative. It seems unlikely, however, that the National Association of Emergency Medical Technicians will detour from its commitments to professionalization. In a sense, if the EMTs and paramedics want to gain greater control over the content of their work, which is not the same as gaining control over the conditions, they will have to achieve the status of what the larger community considers an esteemed occupation. Only then can they obtain the more pervasive, broad-based community-mandated authority and control characteristic of the more established professions.

Recently health-care occupations in the United States have not found it difficult to gain prestige, given our concern with health and well-being. It has not, however, been easy for those in health-care occupations that work directly with patients to abandon the professional alternative and seek occupational advancement exclusively through unionization. Consequently the emergency ambulance worker and paramedic may seek to gain local advancement through a union and continue to seek societal esteem and recognition through professionalization. The success of the medical profession in our society is all too evident to most of those in the health-care occupations and serves to encourage the adoption of the professional alternative.

CONCLUSION

It is difficult to predict the professional future of an occupation established less than fifteen years ago. Yet as prehospital emergency care gets increasing attention in our society, those trained to do emergency ambulance work desire to find their place in the hierarchy of medical-care occupations.

This short chapter has presented the theme that as in any other occupation, emergency ambulance workers are eager to promote their own occupational interests. In particular, they want more recognition and prestige and greater control over the content and conditions of their work. Evidence has been presented that such emergency medical work can be considered an emerging profession. Some of the characteristics of the more established professions are present: advanced educational training, national association, collectivity orientation, and a code of ethics. Each of these characteristics, however, exists in only rudimentary form. The strongest professional feature appears to be a firm commitment toward the patient's interests and well-being.

Unionization is indeed another means for the EMT and paramedic seeking to gain occupational control and authority. Although some might state that the twin processes of unionization and professionalism are contradictory and incompatible, my own argument is that for some occupations, such as emergency ambulance workers, greater control of both the conditions and the content of their work must involve both alternatives.

7

STRESS AND EMERGENCY AMBULANCE WORK

To live in our modern complex world is daily to confront the strains and demands of everyday life. Life in any society presents a series of challenges, trials, and tribulations that human beings must deal with in some way. Most people never really achieve total mastery over these stresses, but rather develop strategies of adaptation that permit some emotional satisfaction and allow them to live a reasonably happy, normal life. For most people, life is filled with petty annoyances and daily irritations here and there punctuated with the more significant of life's stresses, such as the death of a loved one, the loss of job, or a serious illness. Such events call for more significant methods of adaptation, and since they occur less frequently, they are often the most difficult with which to cope and people turn more to others for help.

Within this more universal set of human pressures, there are more specific or limited areas of stress, which are unique because of circumstance or setting—these might include those associated with particular circumstances or events, like marriage and divorce, or special environments like one's place of work, one's community, or some other organizational setting. The kinds of work that people perform present them with a variety of stress-producing situations. Indeed, virtually every occupation has its own strains and demands, its problematic events and circumstances. To perform certain kinds of work requires that a person learn not only the skills and techniques necessary to that occupation but also the strategies for adapting to or coping with the stresses and demands that accompany that particular form of work. Studies in sociology and psychology tell us that not all work presents the same kind of stress; some occupations have relatively low levels of strain

143

associated with them, whereas others are highly stressful and require that those who perform that kind of work adapt to the many and varied forms of strain inherent in their occupation. Social service work is an example of the kind of occupation that places significant stress on those so employed, who must on a daily basis deal with and attempt to solve the myriad trials and tribulations of their clientele. While social service work is acknowledged to be especially stressful, the work performed in emergency situations is even more demanding.[15] In this sense emergency workers, such as police, firemen, and emergency ambulance workers have all the problems associated with being of service to others, but also all the pressures of circumstances of medical emergency that add to the significance of these problems. To understand something about the everyday world of emergency ambulance crews, we must examine the everyday events that make special demands upon the physical and emotional resources of those who choose this kind of work. What follows is an analysis of the routine everyday events of the EMT and paramedic with special emphasis placed on the physically and emotionally problematic features of the work.

STRESS AND THE EMT AND PARAMEDIC

Although EMTs and paramedics confront a variety of stressful conditions in their everyday work, at County Hospital these conditions were seldom talked about directly, for reasons to be made clear later but that became evident to me only in the course of interviews and the bits and pieces of conversation that occurred in the interval between runs.

For the most part, the EMTs and paramedics seemed to regard such strains and stress as a normal part of their work. They tended to view such problems as part of what they must adapt to in order to do the kind of work they had chosen to perform. And indeed they were correct. While there are actually no clear-cut parameters for these stressful conditions, there seem to me to be four particular factors that contribute to the strains inherent in the working life of EMTs and paramedics: the lack of personal time in which to satisfy biological necessities; the uneven nature of emergency work; the dangers and risks associated with ambulance work; the need to confront dead, dying, and critically injured patients as routine everyday events. There is no hierarchy of importance to these problems and the sequence in which they are discussed below in no way implies such an order.

PERSONAL TIME

All human beings must satisfy certain biological requirements if they are to sustain life. Finding the time and opportunity to eat, sleep, rest, and go to the toilet are requirements of daily living that most people face and solve without too much thought. This is especially true of those who are fortunate enough to be in the comfortably controlled environment of their own home. In such organized work settings as offices, factories, and department stores, the problem increases somewhat, but most modern work establishments provide the time, space, and other facilities needed by their employees. Employee cafeterias, lounges, lavatories, and snack bars are all part of most industrial and business organizations, and employees have come to expect these as part of management's obligation to its workers. More important, however, is having the spare time required to carry out these activities. Most working persons require not only the place but also sufficient time to carry out these activities. Industrial and business organizations supply this too, and in fact the rhythms of work in most organizations pulsate around these biological requirements. The temporal working day of employees is structured and regulated around such events as coffee break, rest period, lunchtime, time-out periods to use the bathroom, etc. Employees consider them expected events, relied-upon and even taken-for-granted periods of time to satisfy biological necessities.

For EMTs and paramedics, these expected, anticipated, and even necessary periods of free time do not exist. The time to eat, to relax and rest, to go to the toilet, is highly problematic. It is not that there is no time for these activities, for in fact often there is ample time. The problem is that EMTs and paramedics have no way of knowing when and if they will have the time. They are on duty the moment they clock in at the beginning of the shift. From that moment on, they are responsible for all emergency runs that the dispatcher assigns to them. There is virtually no way to plan for any other events because it is impossible to anticipate when a run will occur. There may be several runs, one after another all morning, and then a complete blank during the afternoon. While EMTs and paramedics take time-out, these time-outs are not formally structured into the work itself, nor can they be regulated into the working time itself. Emergency ambulance crews cannot refuse to take a run because someone is eating, resting, or in the bathroom. An emergency run by its very nature has priority over all such activities. A district ambulance or paramedic unit that is in service must respond to any and every run assigned.

For EMTs and paramedics—and this is the common plight of all emergency workers—whatever opportunities for time and space there are to satisfy private biological needs must be informally created; they cannot be formally structured into the work as organizationally sanctioned, work-interrupted events. Unlike many employees, EMTs and paramedics cannot look forward to a lunch hour or coffee break as a fixed period of time to be counted on and anticipated. For the EMT and paramedic, the workday is filled with examples of interrupted meals and rest periods. Emergency ambulance crews are often called on runs, after having just started breakfast or lunch—often ordered in a diner. A leisurely begun and ended meal with a chance for small talk is an unusual treat for EMTs and paramedics.

While the typical work shift for many emergency ambulance workers is replete with runs and there is much time spent in waiting for one, what might seem to be free time is not really free. It is time that EMTs and paramedics use—and, no doubt, hospital administrations expect them to do so—to eat, relax, and go to the bathroom, but these cannot be relied upon or considered as expected fixed events. Lunches are skipped because of a run; rest periods are violated for the same reason. As a result, EMTs and paramedics often take whatever time and opportunities are available; they snatch at the chance to eat, for example, even though the time and place are far from perfectly matched. Although many people in our society consider noon the appropriate time for lunch, and the evening hour the proper time for dinner, in emergency ambulance work things rarely turn out so neatly. For instance, an ambulance crew may decide to "grab some lunch," not because it is time for lunch—it may be an hour or so before noon—but because the crew is close to a fast-food strip. The assumption is that later, the noon hour, their location may be disadvantageous—no nearby place to eat—or the crew may be in the middle of a run.

As a result, EMT and paramedic crews often find themselves eating at odd hours, skipping one or more meals and stuffing down food in the ambulance on the way to a run. In Metro-City, I saw on many occasions the waste baskets in the district ambulance and paramedic units include among their contents empty coffee cups, half-eaten sandwiches, doughnuts, and rolls, evidence of a run-interrupted breakfast or lunch.

One experienced County Hospital paramedic expressed his feelings this way:

> There's a certain level of tension maintained throughout the shift. Since we get runs at anytime, your meals are interrupted. Even taking a crap, you can't relax.

As significant as this kind of stress is, EMTs and paramedics accept it as part of their work and find ways of adapting to it. In emergency medical work in general and in ambulance work in particular, time is indeed a difficult substance to manage. As stated earlier, it is not that EMTs and paramedics have no time for eating, resting, and so on; but that time is unpredictable, unstable.

One of the ways that EMTs and paramedics adapt to this is to make time for themselves during their shift. In addition to the amount of time spent in the ambulance or the crew room waiting for a run, which crews are expected to make use of for eating and relaxing, there is another form of time that is unlikely to be interrupted by a run. This is the time spent "out of service" in which the crew of an emergency ambulance cannot be called on to respond to a run.

An ambulance crew is considered out of service when their ambulance is in maintenance awaiting vehicle repairs, or when a unit is in the process of responding to a run, e.g., at the scene or in transport to an emergency room. Once a patient has been transported to a hospital emergency room, the dispatcher gives the crew some minutes to take the patient in and provide the doctors and nurses with whatever information about the patient there is available. The dispatcher also assumes that the crew will need time—a few minutes usually—to clean up the ambulance, to wash out the blood and dirt, to rearrange supplies and equipment, to put new sheets on the stretcher cot, and see to other similar details. Because all district ambulances and paramedic units notify the dispatcher via two-way radio when they have arrived at the emergency room— referred to as "marking on the scene"—the dispatcher allows several minutes for the unit to remain out of service at the emergency room in order to complete the run. After several minutes though, the dispatcher expects the crew to "mark back in service" and thus be available for another run. If a crew feels it needs some personal time, however, they will simply delay for several minutes to report that they are back in service.

The County Hospital dispatchers whom I talked to were very much aware of this tactic—many had used it themselves when they were on the street and allowed these time-out efforts to occur. They were very alert, however, to abuses of this informal arrangement, and would not tolerate extended out-of-service periods. If a crew did not report back in service within fifteen or twenty minutes, its members ran the risk of the dispatcher checking on their status and making inquiries about their activities.

One dispatcher who described to me the nuances of this phenomenon remarked:

> I give paramedic units more time out of service at an emergency room because they need to clean up the ambulances after a trauma run or cardiac arrest. If they need more time, all they have to do is call us on the phones.

Here the dispatcher was giving paramedic units the implicit opportunity to take more time for themselves by phoning to request additional time. In this sense, the phone calls legitimize a request for more time.

If it is a slow shift and the dispatcher has no runs to give out to the various crews, he or she may let a unit stay out of service several minutes more than usual. Likewise, there are occasions when the dispatchers are so busy that they ask about the status of an ambulance or paramedic crew almost immediately after their arrival at an emergency room. These latter occasions prevent the crew members from getting some extra free time, but most appear to understand that the dispatcher has little choice if the people who are requesting help are to get it promptly.

Of course, quite often an ambulance crew will report back promptly once they have made their transport to an emergency room, and thus signify they are available for another run. Sometimes a crew may then wait an hour before they get one, although of course they are in service the entire time. But the time that an ambulance crew spends waiting for a run is not as free for personal needs as time out of service. Even time out of service at an emergency room is of limited value, since what the crew members can do is limited. An ambulance crew could never stay out of service long enough to drive to another part of town to eat or run an errand, for example.

Another way EMTs and paramedics learn to cope with the demands of finding time to eat is to dine at carry-out establishments, and some EMTs bring their own home-prepared food to work. Some bring their food in a lunchbox and prepare the kind of meals that can be eaten quickly or periodically sampled during waiting periods. Most EMTs and paramedics whom I observed confined their eating to the fast-food variety and often ate in the ambulance. Sometimes a crew actually ate in a cafeteria or sit-down restaurant. The ever-present hand-held radio, however, sat in the middle of the table, reminding everyone that what had started out as a leisurely dinner might last no more than a few minutes. I observed in these situations that there would usually be some kidding and joking—and even bets taken—about the liklihood of actually being able to finish the meal.

WORK RHYTHM

Most work in an organized setting develops a rhythm of its own, in the sense that the time is structured around certain routine events in which the workday passes. This rhythm allows workers to predict and anticipate what will happen to them while they are at work. This tends to lessen the tensions and anxieties associated with working an an environment that the worker neither owns and controls nor can call home. While such a rhythmic predictability may produce boredom, it is apt to reduce stress and anxiety.

Emergency work, on the other hand, is characterized by a lack of rhythm or at least an uneven rhythm of work in which there is little predictability of impending events. In an earlier chapter, this was couched in terms of uncertainty. Part of the uncertain world of emergency ambulance work is that a crew begins a shift of duty with no idea of what the shift will bring or require. The members of the crew cannot know when they can eat or rest, how much work they will do—how many runs—or even what kind of work they will be called on to perform. Here is an example: once when I was an observer at County with a paramedic unit on the day shift (7:00–3:00), we went the entire morning without a single run and then had three runs during the noon hours (11:30–1:30) when the crew might have expected to eat. The afternoon hours might and often did bring several runs during a short span of time and then no more runs would occur until the second shift took over at 3:00.

It has frequently been observed that periods of lull and quiet are quickly followed by those of intense activity. When will these alternate situations arise? The answer is, no one knows or can predict.

For EMTs and paramedics this creates the tension that is characteristic of their work, in which no one can ever let down or relax because there is no way of knowing what the next few minutes may bring. Most EMTs and paramedics contend that they try to put this sort of tension out of their minds and concentrate on what is at hand. One paramedic had this to say about his feelings:

> I try not to think about it [getting a run]. Unless there is something I'm trying to do. If I've got an errand to run or we're trying to eat, then I don't like runs to interfere. I think of that as my time.
>
> *Observer:* What do you feel when you hear the alert tone?
> *Paramedic:* If it's a gunshot or stabbing—or if we know it's a real bad accident, I get the adrenalin flowing. I really want to get there.

It must, of course, be pointed out that all coping and adaptive strategies to the problematic features of work have their limitations and disadvantages. The adaptive strategies developed by EMTs and paramedics are no exception. The next section will examine some of the mechanisms used to adapt to the uneven rhythms of work in light of the limitations.

There seem to be two important problems associated with the uneven rhythm or lack of predictability in emergency ambulance work. The first is how to fill the lulls or waiting periods with meaningful and enjoyable activity. The second, how to maintain a professional posture during such periods. Although, in a sense, they are two distinct problems; they are also interrelated.

The interconnectedness of these problems was made clear to me in comments made by an experienced paramedic at County:

EMT work is a case of sit on your butt and bust your butt. You wait for hours for something to happen, and all hell breaks loose. It's hard to keep a professional commitment. You get relaxed and let down professionalism, and then things get going and you have to be professional. It would be easier to be busy all the time and be professional all the time.

This paramedic had discovered in his own way the essence of an important problem in the work that EMTs and paramedics do. Without going into the historical details of the development of the work, my own observations seemed to indicate that EMTs and paramedics tend to see themselves as professionals and have hopes of achieving professional status. Their view of a professional worker seems to include training in a particular technique, client service, collective orientation—putting the needs and interests of others ahead of self and maintaining an aura of maturity, responsibility, and self-assurance in the conduct of work. Part of how the EMT and paramedic sees himself or herself as a professional involves conducting their work in a mature, responsible, competent fashion.

In addition to the striving and desires of the EMTs and paramedics themselves for professional status, officials at the ambulance division at County Hospital also encouraged the professionalism of the EMT employees. Administrators in the division take every occasion to exhort and encourage the professionalism of the EMTs, and dress codes and departmental norms of public behavior were strictly enforced. Many of the communications from the ambulance division administration concerning rules and regulations for work appealed to the professional sensibilities of the EMTs and paramedics in adhering to and supporting division policies and regulations. Yet the very nature of ambulance work means that much time must be spent in waiting for runs away from the view of the public, patients, and hospital officials.

Waiting for runs is a period of time that must in some way be filled meaningfully, and there are few opportunities for it to be formally structured or managed, since the availability to make a run must be maintained. Waiting periods are thus filled informally, in accordance with mutually agreed-upon norms and values regarding time. I refer to this informally structured waiting period as a different kind of time-out. This means that it is characterized by a kind of suspended animation in which at least some of the activities engaged in have a kind of "don't really count" quality to them. Much of the behavior is not serious, nor is it meant to be. As I note later in this chapter, such nonserious behavior has adaptive and latent functions. It is a form of tension release.

Much of these time-out periods, we have already observed, is filled with games and play, kidding, joking, and mostly just plain conversation or talk. The language used in conversation is almost always loose, often profane, and since it is spoken backstage—out of view of the public, patients, and hospital officials—the talk often tends to center around the characteristics of and dealings with patients, administrators, and those ambulance crews who are absent. To Eric, the paramedic quoted earlier, this time-out connoted an absence of professional decorum and stance. He tended to view the teasing, kidding, and other nonserious behavior indulged in waiting periods as professionally demeaning and unbecoming. Yet it is well known among medical sociologists that these are common practices among many professional groups during such periods and serve the important function of relieving the tensions and anxieties associated with medical work.

ADAPTING TO THE WORK RHYTHM

The uneven or uncertain rhythms of emergency medical work make periods of waiting for time out all the more important. Whatever time-outs there are must be filled in ways that are meaningful and tension releasing.

Because a good deal of the waiting for a run occurs in the ambulance itself, some crews attempt to personalize the ambulance space—that is, they take space that is essentially neutral, functional, and rather stark (many people no doubt feel uneasy just looking inside an ambulance)—and make it a bit more livable. Attempts to make the ambulance more homelike, or a sort of home territory are ways of making the time spent inside the ambulance more comfortable, enjoyable and bearable.

For example, the paramedic crew on one County Hospital ambulance installed a rather elaborate and expensive stereo system with the speakers mounted on the inside wall of the vehicle. An FM station with continuous rock music was the preferred channel, and this stream of music provided the background for those periods of time when the crew was waiting for a run. The members of its crew were proud of this installation and called it to my attention more than once.

On still another occasion at County during the approach of the cold winter months, a paramedic crew spent several hours during the day shift searching stores for a space heater, which was to be mounted in the rear compartment of their ambulance. The crew was concerned that many of the drugs and medications they carried would freeze with prolonged exposure to the cold, and the space heater would prevent this and provide additional warmth when needed. After an appropriate heater was found, there were fairly elaborate designs drawn up to see how the unit could best be mounted. This seems to demonstrate the personalized care that ambulance crews give their vehicles, which goes far beyond routine mechanical maintenance. In living space, the vehicles are made to feel like home, and the articles housed in the vehicle are given the kind of care and attention that people give to objects in their homes. Here the ambulance space is no longer neutral; it is not simply a vehicle to drive or a place to work in. It is lived in. It is the space in which time is spent and passed, conversations held, and past events relived. For these reasons and others, ambulance crews consider the space deserves to be personalized and upgraded to something almost approaching the importance of home.

There are other attempts and strategies to fill waiting time with what is considered useful and meaningful activities. The start of each shift—7:00, 3:00, and 11:00—is usually a kind of adjustment period for the new crew going on duty. Normally the EMTs and paramedics will check the supplies in their vehicle—especially the medical supplies—and will busy themselves restocking whatever supplies and equipment are lacking. The checking is never done hurriedly but methodically and slowly, as if the entire day or evening might be given over to this activity. Also during this period when those on the shift are just starting and provided that there is no run to which they must respond, the crew will discuss any errands that someone may want to do. The difficulty, of course, here is that whatever one member of a crew wants to do his or her partner, or all the members of a paramedic crew, must do also. Normally, whatever claims to a particular errand are made by one crew member, the others feel bound to honor. If the beginning of the shift starts slowly, without a run, the errands may be taken care of immediately.

For members of the more experienced EMT and paramedic crews at County Hospital, the waiting time might be filled in by a visit to a "favorite spot." The EMTs and paramedics had come to know Metro-City very well, and in each district the crews had a number of favored settings in which to spend some time. These settings included certain magazine stands, short-order cafes, and carry-out shops. And over the months and years, the crews had come to know well the clerks, waitresses, and others who worked in these places. Their relationships had become personal, close, and at times intimate—many times on a first-name basis. It was a favorable arrangement for both parties. The clerks and waitresses needed the business, and the emergency ambulance crews needed the place to be in, to hang out, and to find in it someone to talk to.

During the winter months, the crew room at County and the crew rooms at the other emergency hospital stations in Metro-City were the places most used for activities to fill waiting time. They also became personalized spaces with cartoons posted on bulletin boards, and other small additions to make them appear more homelike. Whatever time was spent there was usually given over to conversation, games, kidding, and other forms of horseplay. The manifest function of all this activity was to pass the time between runs. The latent function had to do with testing commitments to certain values and meanings associated with emergency ambulance work, the discussion of which is reserved for later.

ACCEPTING RISKS AND DANGER

EMTs and paramedics face many situations of risk and danger in the course of their work, and this constitutes the second problematic and stressful feature associated with the occupation. Doing emergency ambulance work can be and often is dangerous to the health and safety of those thus employed. It is a risky business, and the risks taken have several forms. The most common everyday risk taken is the driving to an emergency scene at high speed. Other risks that are taken less frequently but often enough encountered are the dangers associated with scenes of crime, domestic violence, fire, and explosion.

EMTs and paramedics consider response time—the time an ambulance takes to get to the scene of the emergency—highly important. Getting to an emergency victim quickly, in a matter of minutes, is often crucial in a patient's ability to survive or recover. As a result, all runs are responded to with speed. EMTs do not always use the highest speed possible—this is reserved for only certain runs—but they do use speeds far in excess of posted speed limits. In responding to an emergency, a speed of from 60 to 70 on city streets is common. On a crosstown expressway the speed often approaches or exceeds 90 mph.

The EMTs and paramedics at County recognized the risks and dangers of driving at such high speeds, but they rarely discussed those aspects of their work—unless prodded by the researcher. When I asked them about such speedy driving, most opened up and admitted that it was something they often thought about, but had learned to accept and live with. In the words of one EMT:

> Ambulance work is more risky than police or fire because we have more runs and go red lights and siren [speed] to every run.

Every run that an ambulance crew responds to is considered an emergency; the driver always uses red lights and siren, and speeds in getting to the scene. There are occasions when the ambulance itself is involved in an accident en route to a scene or in transport with a patient. During the year prior to this particular study, a paramedic from County was critically injured in an accident en route to the scene, and during the course of my own research, there were several accidents involving County Hospital vehicles. No one in the ambulance was killed or critically injured, but several of them were badly enough injured to have to remain home for some time.

According to one EMT whom I interviewed, a rookie EMT is considered the most dangerous driver to ride with. This EMT felt that being a good driver can only come by gaining experience and knowing the terrain and the limitations of one's own vehicle. Such knowledge takes time to acquire, and there is a distinct learning process involved. This EMT in the course of our conversation mentioned that the new partner he was working with made him feel very uncomfortable when he drove.

As in all types of work, EMTs and paramedics take pride in possessing certain skills and abilities, and driving an ambulance at a very high rate of speed is a source of pride to some. One afternoon, while I was an observer at County Hospital on a run that took us to a truck accident on an interstate expressway, the following incident took place:

> On the way to the scene the paramedic who was driving, was driving very fast on the expressway, and an EMT who was riding in the rear compartment with me remarked to the driver "And you thought I was crazy!"

After the run was completed, the paramedic who was driving told me that when the call for an ambulance came in, the dispatcher sent two other units to the scene two minutes before sending ours. The paramedic said that he wanted to be first on the scene even though we were two minutes behind: "It would have been real shitty if we hadn't been first to get there." We were, indeed the first unit on the scene.

Another EMT told me that paramedic ambulance units always travel at breakneck speed since it is assumed that every run is a life-threatening emergency. District ambulance units use more discretion and do not drive at the fastest rate possible on some runs. This EMT also went on to say:

> Driving fast is not the same as driving reckless. If a driver goes at fifty miles per hour through a red light, that's reckless. He's asking for trouble.

While all ambulance units—district ambulances and paramedic units alike—respond to a run with red lights and siren, they do not always transport that way. When a patient is being transported to the hospital, EMTs and paramedics believe that fast driving increases the danger for the patient, as well as adding to the patient's fears and anxieties about being in an ambulance. Since district ambulances do not transport the critically ill or injured, they rarely transport with speed. The paramedic units, however, transport only the critical patients and must exercise judgment about the speed at which they travel to an emergency room. Since paramedics give their patients more definitive medical care, the patient's condition is normally stabilized before transport, and there is less need to drive at high speed. Often the paramedic unit will transport a patient at the legally prescribed speed, traveling without red lights and siren. If they decide to increase speed of transport, the paramedics will tell the driver to travel at "easy ten" which means that the driver will use red lights and siren to cross intersections but maintain normal posted speed. On those occasions, however, when the paramedics have been unable to stabilize the patient's condition and the patient is near death, the unit will travel at "signal ten," which is top speed, using red lights and siren. In such cases, it is assumed the patient has only minutes to live and requires the immediate attention of an emergency-room facility.

Many paramedic units transport patients at easy ten and the ambulance proceeds with the legally prescribed rate of speed. The following interchange took place when the prescribed speed was not maintained.

> *Paramedic A:* The other night I couldn't get Willie [the EMT driver] to slow down. We had a patient in the ambulance and I asked Willie for an easy ten. I looked up at one point, and Willie was doing fullboard on the expressway! Has he been on vacation?

Paramedic B: Yes, he just got off.

Paramedic A: I quess that's it. He's full of adrenaline.

Here Paramedic A explains the EMT driver's disregard of the "easy-ten" request as due to the energy (adrenaline) obtained from a vacation rest. The assumption is that vacations energize EMTs, and they respond by driving too fast. In this case there was a violation of the driving norms and a corresponding explanation of the deviance. One of the ways that EMTs and paramedics cope with the risks of high-speed driving is to try to assure themselves that no ambulance driver goes faster than is necessary. This is not always easy to do, and I turn to the discussion of it now.

COPING WITH DRIVING RISKS

As with other forms of stress, emergency ambulance crews develop a variety of psychological mechanisms to cope with the anxiety of having an accident because they must daily drive at so high a speed. The most common form is acceptance, as the paramedics and EMTs attempt to remove such thoughts and fears from consciousness. As one EMT remarked:

The first few days as an EMT I was scared to death! But you get used to it.

Getting used to it though is not enough. There must be a rationalization for removing such fears from consciousness. One such rationalization is trust. Quite simply EMTs and paramedics learn to trust the person who is doing the driving. Because ambulance crews often take turns driving, learning to trust one's self is part of this process too. The County Hospital EMTs and paramedics often discussed the shortcomings of other drivers who did not "measure up" to their own driver. Because this favorable reaction to their own driver was repeated to me by different crews, it would appear that a prevalent way of coping with the risks of driving at so high a rate of speed is to have implicit trust in your own driver. None of them could say for certain why their driver was good, and the drivers of other units not as good. It was as if they must convince themselves that their driver was someone they could trust if they were to be able to do their work without thinking of the risks involved.

Not all ambulance drivers, however, are trusted, and at least one veteran paramedic recalled a driver with whom he found it impossible to work:

I trust them, but there have been some I didn't trust. If they get too bad, I'll get a hold of the supervisor and make him aware of the problem. I remember one guy though that had a habit that once he got a run, he had only two speeds. That was as fast as he could go and faster! That guy actually scared me to death! He had no control of the ambulance—he just kind of stampeded it.

Another form of coping is what the EMTs call "defensive driving." One EMT defined this and talked about this value:

I drive defensively. I assume the other drivers on the street [non-emergency drivers] are bad drivers and will make mistakes. I anticipate that others are going to be careless. Also I believe in the safety of the ambulance. They're safer at high speed than my own car.

For this EMT, defensive posturing is considered vital in a world of careless drivers, and the element of trust is extended to the vehicle as well. The County ambulance division administration also believes in the efficacy of defensive driving: one of the bulletin boards in the main office is adorned with a poster that reads "Defensive Driving Can Save Your Life."

EMTs and paramedics do their work in a world of fleeting encounters and ever-present risks and dangers. As a result they tend to develop an implicit trust in what in their working world is closest to them, such as their own driver, their own ambulance. Although they do not always know *why* they trust the driver of their vehicle, they need this confidence in order to work. Until events prove otherwise—a driver proves unsafe, or their vehicle fails to respond—that implicit trust remains manifest. By the same token there is an implicit distrust in whatever is outside their immediate world; other drivers in other vehicles face threats just by being "out there." Even other emergency vehicles cannot be trusted; as one EMT remarked:

One of my greatest fears is that someday I'm going to be wiped out by another goddamn emergency ambulance.

There is yet another important strategy for coping with the risks of ambulance riding and that takes the form of interpersonal kidding and teasing among the crews. In a study a few years ago of high-steel workers, the sociologist Jack Haas discovered that men who work on high steel do a lot of kidding and teasing of each other to test how much a given person in a dangerous place might be trusted.[16] Confidence in one's co-workers is an important feature among high-steel workers, and those who can take teasing without getting upset or defensive, are considered worthy of trust. Those who cannot take teasing cannot be counted on to keep their cool in risky high-steel situations. My own personal observation showed that EMTs and paramedics also kid and tease one another, and it is certainly arguable that this serves the same function as it does for Haas's high-steel workers.

Much of the teasing among ambulance crews centers around a person's driving ability which seems to indicate that this is considered a risky hidden dimension of their work and that there is a need to test the trustworthiness of the driver. The following personal anecdotes exemplify some of this reaction:

> Several EMTs were chatting with an emergency-room nurse about physical exercise. One of them stated that "to get effective exercise you have to produce a pulse rate of one hundred and twenty for at least one half hour three days a week."
>
> One of the paramedics in the crew quickly remarked, "I don't have to do that—I get that effect everytime John drives!"

> We were in a paramedic unit proceeding down the expressway en route to an accident scene. At a high rate of speed—90 mph—the driver maneuvered the ambulance between a car and a truck. The paramedic in the rear compartment with me winced and yelled to the others in the front seat, "Hey, we better check Dale's chauffeur's license!"

OTHER DANGERS

Yet another category of risks is associated with the emergency scenes themselves. EMTs and paramedics are sent to scenes of violence and crime in order to provide life support for the injured involved. This often places the ambulance crew in a dangerous situation because often the crime is still virtually going on. A good response time can mean that the ambulance crew reaches the scene more quickly than the police and that the perpetrators of the crime may still be on the scene. An experienced paramedic describes a situation that he confronted:

> We got a call from dispatch about a man shot and the address was just two or three blocks from where we happened to be. We got there before the police or anybody. I ran inside, and there lay a guy shot six times in the chest—but alive. When I leaned over him to start patching him up, I felt something poking me in the back of the neck. I turned around to see what it was, and it was the guy who shot him still holding the pistol. He said, "Is he going to live or will he die?" I said, "Buddy, if I can help it he's going to live." And he said, "That's all I wanted to know," and he ran out the back door and I ran out the front door! I didn't go back in until the police got there and when we went in—the guy on the floor was dead.

This paramedic was "rewarded" for his good response time by almost becoming a victim himself.

As many police know, domestic disturbances can be one of the most dangerous encounters in all law enforcement. EMTs and paramedics face the same problems, and they have little way of knowing whether they will confront a violent scene or not. Very often when they are summoned to assist someone at home, the situation turns out to be dangerous without there having been any warning or foreknowledge.

A paramedic at County Hospital described for me an experience that occurred during the day shift:

> We got into the house where the dispatcher told us to find a sick person. A lady took us down the hall to a bedroom, and she told us to go in and get her husband because he had to go to the hospital. As we walked in, we were looking down the barrel of a big revolver, and the man in bed, pointing it at us, said, "I want you guys to leave me alone. I'm not going anywhere." I answered him with "That's fine with me—we're leaving."
>
> So we backed out and started down the hall. The wife came up and said, "No, no, you can't leave him. He's got to go to the hospital. The doctor's already signed the papers. He's a little silly in the head. I'll go get the gun and you can go in!" She came out and said, "It's OK now."
>
> We walked in, and he reached under the pillow and pulled out another gun and said, "I told you to get the hell out of here. Now leave me alone!" Before we could get to the front door the wife had the second gun and said, "It's OK now, these are the only guns he has." We entered again, and he reached under the bed and pulled out a third gun she didn't know he had! He threatened to blow our brains out if we didn't get out of there—so we left.

There are times, of course, when the EMTs and paramedics respond to emergency scenes with the police and can count on the protection of the police who accompany them. While often this serves to dissuade people from threatening harm to the ambulance crew, there are times when even a police escort is not effective in warding off potential danger. A paramedic at County remembered an experience of this nature:

> We had a call for a man cut. Got to the scene same time as the police did, and I was first one in the door. When I opened the door and stepped inside, the lady who stabbed the man still had a butcher knife in her hand, and she arced it through the air at me and just missed my throat by inches. The victim was lying on the couch just cut to pieces. The police had to go in and restrain her before

we could go back in. She was really going to nail whoever walked through that door. And I just happened to be the first one inside.

The EMTs and paramedics in Metro-City, especially those who had had some street experience, considered certain areas and certain commercial locations in Metro-City more dangerous than others. Working-class and lower-class bars, poolrooms, and other hangouts in poverty-stricken areas were considered unsafe places to go to on a run, particularly on the second and third shift. While the inner-city areas or tenement districts of Metro-City supply the ambulance division with a sizable number of its runs, they are considered risky because of the violence that is one of the characteristics of these areas. One paramedic with several years' experience on the street had these thoughts about the dangerous areas of Metro-City:

Anytime we get runs to the housing projects in the summertime, it's always dangerous—not as bad though as in 1973 and 1974. We used to have orders not to go into any housing projects without a police escort. They [residents] threw bricks at us, beer bottles, wine bottles. We would get surrounded by about a hundred people, and they would rock the ambulance. Hell, they would do that to the firemen too.

Despite the risks and dangers involved in going into those sections of the city noted for conflict and violence, there is little that the EMTs and paramedics at County can do about it. No run to any address can be refused, and the responding ambulance crew can do little more than hope that the police will be on the scene too, or that in any event they can do their work and depart in peace. Most EMTs felt that this was an aspect of their work over which they had little control; they simply accepted the fact and thereby learned to live with it.

WORKING WITH THE DYING AND DEAD

EMTs and paramedics confront as everyday events some of the most tragic human circumstances. Virtually each day, they see people dying because of heart attacks, poisonings, shootings, stabbings, and other forms of violent accidents. They work on patients injured in automobile wrecks who are not only traumatically injured but often unrecognizably mutilated and disfigured. They administer to fire victims whose bodies are charred and wracked with excruciating pain. They treat children afflicted by a variety of perils—from those severely sick and injured to those abused and neglected. Since ambulance workers are generally the first medical-care personnel on the scene, they routinely witness the stark realities of human pain and trauma, people with bodies still bleeding, whose suffering is yet to be numbed by drugs, whose mutilated and traumatized bodies are yet to be covered up, sewn up, or treated in some way that will make them "look better." Whatever horrors human existence has to offer by way of disease, accident, violence, and neglect, EMTs and paramedics confront as daily occurrences and first-hand witnessed events.

Yet their work requires them to carry out their medical routines as if it were a classroom exercise. Those they work for and those they treat expect them to deliver the techniques and skills of life support in a cool, calm, efficient, and swift manner. They are there to stabilize the patient's condition and to transport. One only has to read the newspapers or watch the evening TV news to see the coverage of the day's tragedies, and usually there is an ambulance in the background.

Medical sociologists have described the problem that health-care workers have in maintaining a sufficiently detached concern when treating and working with patients.[17] Basically the problem for health-care workers is one of retaining a sense of objectivity toward a patient's condition so that the canons of medical science can be applied to the signs and symptoms manifested by the patient. The health-care professional is also, however, expected to give the patient emotional support or empathy, recognizing the humanity and individual uniqueness of the patient. This is a difficult stance to take requiring a delicate balance between objectivity and subjectivity. According to researchers, the dilemma is so basic to medical practice that doctors and nurses learn this attitude early in the course of their medical education.

The EMTs and paramedics at County Hospital are faced with the same problem in a slightly different way. They spend only a relatively few minutes with their patients and therefore there is little time to develop emotional ties with them. As human beings, however, they cannot be indifferent toward or oblivious to the human suffering and tragedy which they daily witness. They are trained to be objective and detached in giving basic and advanced life support. Yet the subjective or emotional component of their work is something that must be coped with as well. EMTs and paramedics have developed several ways of dealing with the daily rigors of working with the dying and critically ill. These strategies are worth examining.

COPING

EMTs and paramedics cannot fail to be concerned with the suffering of their patients, but they cannot allow that concern to interfere with their ability to give objective, technical emergency care. The most basic device that emergency ambulance crews use in doing their work is a very common one among health-care workers—suppression of emotion. This is referred to in various ways as "putting it out of your mind," or "trying not to think about it." However it is phrased, the process involves removing the "affective" or emotional dimension of what was witnessed from consciousness. To put it another way, it means a narrowing concentration on only the immediate situation or events at hand.

EMTs and paramedics make their work easier by concentrating mechanically and methodically on the single aspect of the patient's being that they feel they are best trained to deal with—the physical manifestations of illness or injury. According to one paramedic:

> You cover up your emotions to get the job done. Try not to think about what is happening. Later the reality of what happened hits you.

Still another experienced paramedic expressed it in this way:

> I don't let my emotions interfere with my work. If you feel the same things that the patient does, you can't do your job. After it's over, you talk about it, and what happened begins to sink in.

And finally a third paramedic refers to the ability to concentrate on the "immediate" things and the blocking-out of those aspects of the scene he is not prepared to deal with:

> I think about how bad something is, but I don't dwell on it. It's there, and it's gone just like that. The thing I concentrate on, and I lose track of everything else going on around me, is that I want to help that person and ease that suffering. I can't stand to see it anymore than anyone else. I just don't think about it. I get so engrossed in trying to do what I've been trained to do, I don't think about it.

If the emotional aspects of a tragic scene are suppressed, it is only temporary. The emotional reaction to a patient's pain, injury, death, or other debilitation is blocked out for only a limited period of time. Later the event is reacted to. Usually this comes during time-out periods while waiting for a run. Whether an ambulance crew is waiting in the crew room or in the ambulance, the talk centers around the event. What was seen, felt, experienced, and feared comes out into consciousness in the form of shoptalk. Each person has something to contribute, giving his or her own reactions and feelings about what happened. In a certain sense, without this catharsis, the event or run is incomplete. Only one part has been accomplished—the detached, objective response to a medical emergency. The patient has been administered to and transported to a hospital emergency room, but the event is not over until it has been "talked through." It is not merely the reliving of the event; it is not daydreaming about what might have occurred. It is a way of closing the case, as an ambulance crew's pent-up emotional responses are given their due in the form of talk.

As an observer I often spent hours sitting in the crew rooms, so that there was ample opportunity to hear accounts of the various runs a crew had that day or a day or so previously. Each person had his or her own contribution to make in reconstructing the scene in an attempt to come to terms with what the facts had been. The following conversation took place between two paramedics who were sitting in their ambulance discussing a run they had been on a few days before. The patient, a young male, had had a leg severed in a motorcycle accident.

Paramedic A: I heard they had to cut off his other leg too.

Paramedic B: Yeah, and an arm too.

Paramedic A: He's full of gangrene, but I guess he came out of the coma. The gangrene was caused by the operation and not the result of his accident.

Paramedic A [a few minutes later]: I'm not surprised that he's still alive. He seemed like he had a lot of guts. *[to the researcher]* "He was conscious at the scene and knew his leg was cut off. When we got there, he said he knew he would be in a wheelchair the rest of his life but it wouldn't get him down."

Paramedic B [to the researcher]: I knew the guy! Saw him the week before. Sure didn't think the next time I saw him, he'd be in that condition.

Some EMTs and paramedics take their accounts home with them and use their families as an audience. Just as an office manager recites the "happenings of the day" at home, so some EMTs and paramedics give a rundown of the day's events. While this seems to work for some, there are limitations to this kind of outlet. The details of some stories are too gruesome to be taken home.

A paramedic was describing to me one afternoon two of the runs he had been on the day before. Both had been traumatic runs, and in describing one involving a young child struck by an auto, he exclaimed, "Pretty bad! I don't even tell my wife about those."

Another paramedic I talked with did not think that very many EMTs and paramedics took their day's work home with them:

No, I don't think they do—because they [the family members] can't relate to it. We're the helpers, but who do we turn to for help? We can talk to each other about runs and get the anxiety out of the way. You can't get the same level of feeling across to your family because they don't know what it's like. You might tell them, but you can't explain it to them.

For this paramedic, only his colleagues can really feel what he as an individual feels. There is a "consciousness of kind" here that clearly defines those who "know what it's like" in a direct, experienced sense from those who might listen but cannot really understand.

EMTs and paramedics also cope with the more tragic cases by depersonalizing their relationship with the patient. If a patient and paramedic develop a close interpersonal bond then the paramedic may lose detachment and objectivity and begin to share in the patient's suffering. Although EMTs and paramedics have the opportunity to know the names of the patients they help, they seldom take the time to learn them. When the run is complete, the run sheet or log must also be completed, and the EMT or paramedic responsible must put the patient's name on it. At the scene whoever is handling the run sheet obtains the patient's name in the process of getting other information. My own observation showed that the other EMTs and paramedics often made no attempt to learn the patient's name nor use it in communicating with them. Occasionally the patient's name would be used but with the wrong first name. Often after a patient had been transported to an emergency room, the emergency-room nurse or physician would ask the name of the patient. Usually the EMT or paramedic would have to get the run sheet from his or her partner and read the name of the patient off it.

> One evening the paramedic unit I was observing brought in a young girl injured in an auto accident. The young girl was unconscious, and the paramedics had worked diligently on her at the scene and in transport. When they wheeled her quickly into the emergency room, the doctor said, "What's her name?" One of the paramedics said, "I have no idea."

One paramedic said that the name of a patient stands in low priority compared to other information about the patient that the paramedic feels he or she needs and considered important. Another paramedic commented:

> First things first. Our first priority on a run, if it's anything serious, is to take care of the illness or injury. The name is minor. When I look at a human being lying there, I see the illness or the injury. I don't see John Doe or Mary Doe. I don't care about their life history. I just want to treat that illness or that injury.

The nameless patient remains an object, and this lessens the chance that a more intimate bond between patient and EMT or paramedic will develop. It is more difficult to attach oneself to something or someone that has no name. In this sense a name connotes personalization; it signifies subjective attachment. EMTs and paramedics must remain detached; they cling to their sense of objectivity by leaving their patients nameless.

There are exceptions to this phenomenon, however. There seem to be occasions when EMTs and paramedics want to be able to use a patient's name. This appears to be the case when they want to evoke cooperative behavior from the patient. If an EMT or paramedic is having difficulty eliciting information from a patient, or if the patient acts disoriented, or disturbed enough to interfere with the work of the crew, an EMT or paramedic might use the patient's name in an effort to soothe or calm him or her.

In that case, using a patient's name is manipulative. It is not intended to upgrade the relationship to a personal or primary relationship, but to cajole the patient into a more complying stance. "People we need to communicate with and get on a trusting basis—we get their name. If I can get on a first-name basis, then sometimes things go a lot smoother," an experienced paramedic explained.

There is a sense of detachment, however, even about a named patient because once the name has been learned it is generally quickly forgotten. One EMT who felt this was true said:

I can ask them [the patient] their name, but five minutes after the run is over I couldn't tell you their name. After the run is over, I've completely forgotten it.

The unnamed patients are also more quickly forgotten, it seems. EMTs and paramedics tend to forget events and cases within a few days after they occur unless the run is unusual or considered very serious. The following serves as an example:

One evening I was riding with the same paramedic unit I had ridden with a few weeks earlier. On the prior occasion we had had two traumatic runs that were significant enough to result in media coverage.

I asked one of the paramedics if he had found out what happened to the patients. He remarked that he didn't remember the runs. I said that the runs bothered me so, I had trouble sleeping that night. The paramedic said, "You have to leave it at the hospital. You can't take it home with you."

When I asked the other paramedic on the crew if he remembered the runs, he said, "I don't remember any of it. Just another slab of meat. At home I work on wood—here I work on flesh. It's all the same to me."

This comment was delivered with a smile, and his paramedic partner said, "Ralph, you are cold."

Seeing the patient as an object is an attempt to reduce the humanity of the patient, if not eliminate it entirely, while the EMTs or paramedics are working. It is not that the patient is thought to be nothing more than an object; it is rather that the patient is regarded "as though" he or she were an object. It is a pretense EMTs and paramedics engage in when they are faced with the more severe cases. Otherwise they feel they cannot work.

An experienced paramedic explained:

> In trauma or cardiac arrests you can't look at the patient as a suffering human being—you must look at them as a machine. If it is a myocardal infarct, then it's an electrical pump that's broken down. If the patient is in arrest [cardiac], you get the pump going again.

In this sense the EMT or paramedic plays the role of a mechanic working on a machine that is temporarily out of order. Since a machine neither thinks nor feels, the affective dimension of the work can be overlooked. One need not become emotionally involved with an object that has no emotions, nor show concern for something incapable of suffering.

Still another way that EMTs and paramedics use to cope with the death and dying they routinely see is to take a special interest in those cases that are successfully handled. The essential purpose of the EMT and paramedic is to provide basic and advanced life support. Despite the fact that many patients die, either at the scene, en route to the hospital, or in the emergency room, some patients do indeed recover from critical illnesses or injuries. Their successful recovery is due in part to the life-support care they received at the scene and en route to the hospital. When EMTs and paramedics are successful in helping someone in critical condition to recover, it becomes for them a source of pride and satisfaction.

When a patient in cardiac arrest is successfully resuscitated and lives long enough to be admitted to the hospital and eventually released, EMTs and paramedics refer to this as a "save." Saves are pointed to with much satisfaction, and they are remembered for some time. It is an event worth noting and boasting about in the crew room. These cases seem to be so important that they justify the many stresses associated with emergency medical work, and serve to reenergize an ambulance crew. The following serves as an illustration.

> One of the paramedics I was observing mentioned having free tickets to an upcoming sports event in the city. When I asked how he got free tickets, he said that last year one of the promoters of

the sport had suffered a cardiac arrest—and his paramedic team had resuscitated him.

The paramedic said the man was so grateful he gave the paramedics in the crew free tickets to certain sports events during the year. His paramedic partner told me they visit this person in his home sometimes if they are in the neighborhood, since he is one of their more notable saves.

Other patients are also followed up on to see what kinds of progress the person is making if an ambulance crew was instrumental in helping them in critical condition survive. This does not include all the critical cases, as mentioned earlier, but only the more unusual ones or those where a patient survived when no one expected he or she would do so. In the illustration given earlier about the two paramedics conversing about a patient with a severed leg, the paramedics had elicited from a nurse at the hospital the information about the patient and his subsequent surgery. They followed the patient's recovery for several weeks and continued to check on him even months later.

These cases are relived in conversation, and are considered among the events that make ambulance work worthwhile. I refer to them as "mission-relevant" cases since they signify for EMTs and paramedics some of their best efforts and finest hours.

There are some sorts of runs that serve to justify the problematic features of EMT-paramedic work. They also stand out as good runs because they make bad runs more easy to deal with or live with. A County Hospital paramedic described to me one such run that made him feel good about this work:

> To me, delivering a kid is better than a save, I guess. Because we deal in death, disfigurement, dismemberment so much—my God, it's great to bring something into the world that's new and full of life instead of death. The joy infects everybody. Everyone gets swept up in it.

This brings us to the last coping device to be discussed here. Among saves and births, there are other occurrences that EMTs and paramedics become aware of and that serve to support them in their work. These are the times when private citizens or organizations make some display of appreciation for the efforts of an emergency ambulance crew beyond paying their bill. From time to time the ambulance division at County Hospital receives a handwritten thank-you note from the family or relatives of a patient treated by one of the crews. These notes contain words of thanks and appreciation for the efforts of the persons in that crew. Sometimes the patient was successfully resuscitated; on other occasions, the patient died. Nevertheless, it seems the family was sufficiently impressed with the work of the ambulance crew to send a letter of appreciation. When these cards are received, they are prominently displayed on the bulletin board in the offices of the ambulance division. Sometimes the names of the crew are listed alongside the card if the writer did not include them.

The fact that these notes are always displayed and noticed signifies their importance to the ambulance workers, and this was further borne out by the following personal anecdote:

> Once one of the paramedics whom I was observing showed me a card that he had received in the mail that day. It was a card of appreciation from a woman whose husband had died, but the EMT-paramedic crew had worked very hard to save him. In the card the woman expressed thanks for all the crew had done. The paramedic pointed to the card and said, "This is the only reason why we work."

BURNOUT

In recent years some attention has been given to the phenomenon of burnout among social service workers. Indeed during my own field work at County Hospital several of the more experienced EMTs and paramedics indicated to me they felt "burned out" in their work. When I prodded them, they said that they no longer felt like working, the rewards and satisfactions had disappeared, and with each day, it was increasingly difficult for them to get up for work.

A considerable amount of research has lately been devoted to the problem of burnout, and some interesting patterns have emerged that have bearing on emergency ambulance work. Freudenberger has argued that those most prone to burnout are the dedicated and committed.[18] Since, as we have seen, the work continually demands that EMTs and paramedics must daily risk personal injury, in order to help others, the potential for eventual burnout could indeed be high. Maslach and Pines, the leading researchers in this field, have defined burnout as a loss of concern for people with whom one is working.[19] Among the workers they studied, burnout seems to result from heavy case loads, fatigue, and the lack of structured opportunities for rest and relaxation. These findings have significant implications for EMTs and paramedics, who often must contend with constant runs and, lacking the absence of any formally structured periods of rest, no doubt suffer from fatigue.

McSwain and Shelton in a theoretical article have argued that there are no clearly defined reasons for burnout among EMTs and paramedics; but that the problem is real just the same. The following is from their recent work on this issue:

> The loss of trained emergency medical technicians [EMTs] has been reported variously up to 40 percent in from two to five years. This phenomenon has produced cries of too much work and lack of dedication, continuing education and medical control. Are these reasons or merely excuses why a system does not work as was originally expected? Do individuals become frustrated and fed up with their jobs? Is this because of the bureaucracy under which they work, because they are tired of treating patients who show no appreciation, because they are tired of going into low socio-economic areas where they are at risk of bodily harm, because of the continued pressure, 24-hour days or long shifts without rest? Or is it merely a realization that they are in a field with no future?[20]

The fact that these researchers are so perplexed exemplifies the confusion on the subject of burnout among EMTs and paramedics. While there are some explanations that are more plausible than others, in the following discussion, the conclusions advanced are only tentative. My own personal observations and interviews at County Hospital revealed that the feelings associated with burnout are vague and not clearly explainable to outsiders. An EMT or paramedic would admit to me that he or she felt burned out but would be unable to pinpoint the reason or identify the exact emotions, attitudes, and states of mind that accompanied this feeling.

Several factors, however, seem to be involved. The factor of upward mobility seemed to be important but never completely paramount. Being an EMT or paramedic is certainly for most an occupation with few opportunities for advancement. Although many EMTs and paramedics have college degrees, many others do not, and as they reach the early thirties, where the physical demands of the work begin to take their toll, they look for a way to move up in the ranks into a less physically demanding position. Unfortunately at County Hospital what few administrative positions are available—operations management, education and training, communications—require advanced education and specialized training, and thus are open to only a limited number of EMTs and paramedics. Of course, moving into such medical specialization such as becoming a doctor or nurse is virtually impossible for someone in their thirties and forties.

Coping with the administrative bureaucracy also seems to be connected with the problem of burnout. EMTs and paramedics are street workers and are motivated by the freedom, autonomy, and excitement that emergency medical work offers them. They become accustomed to and learn to expect a certain sense of independence in the performance of their duties, since they work outside the confines of the hospital bureaucracy. Much of their work is carried out with little or no direct supervision, and the rules they must follow tend to be informal and loosely applied. Yet it is the function and destiny of any administrative bureaucracy to create impersonal rules and develop policies and procedures whenever possible. Since the role of the EMT and paramedic is less than fifteen years old, much of their work remains ad hoc, with a minimum of formal policy. As more and more becomes known, however, about the techniques of emergency medicine, it becomes increasingly possible to eliminate the ad hoc nature of the work and to substitute more formal procedures. In short, the discretionary powers of the emergency ambulance worker are beginning to shrink as the administrative bureaucracy increasingly fixes set policies and publishes procedure manuals. For many experienced paramedics, this causes resentment and frustration. Sensing a loss of freedom and autonomy in their work, they become ever more aware of the encroachment of the administrative bureaucracy in their working life. This can and does become a factor in the burnout of those EMTs and paramedics who are the most sensitive to this issue. They talked longingly of the good old days when not everything was done by the book, and they were not constantly receiving memorandums from the office.

The most important factor in burnout among EMTs and paramedics may well be a growing inability to cope with the social-psychological pressures of emergency work. As we have seen, their world is full of danger, risk, human tragedy, and pressure-filled medical judgments. It is a world of life-and-death decisions, caring for the dying, the mutilated, the battered and abused. The normal human emotions are suppressed so that efficient, speedy, and detached medical care can be given. Virtually every day the EMT and paramedic must confront the battleground of the metropolitan milieu: fires, explosions, accidents, shootings, stabbings, and other assorted human misfortunes. If one of the central modes of adaptation or adjustment to this is the suppression of emotion how long can it be maintained? As Maslach and Pines have found, one of the signs of burnout involves the inability of persons to handle their emotions, to the point where the work is no longer tolerable. With few opportunities to move up eventually into the medical hierarchy, to get off the street and behind the desk, how many EMTs and paramedics can continue to work well into their thirties or forties?

The answer seems to be, very few. Eventually the pressures become too great; the emotions can no longer be so readily suppressed; the dangers and risks blocked from consciousness. The job becomes too much, asking more from persons who find that their capacity for increased giving is severely diminished.

> *Researcher:* How do you feel about the stresses that go with your job?
>
> *Eric:* I came home tonight and told my wife I was so depressed I couldn't cope with the work anymore. The older I get, the more it gets to me.
>
> *Researcher:* What is it that's getting to you?
>
> *Eric:* I think the job is finally getting to me. As I get older, my values change. I'm not as reckless as I used to be. I think more of my own mortality. I see death every day or disfigurement—and that makes me aware of my own mortality.
>
> *Researcher:* Do you think it affects others at County too?
>
> *Eric:* It burns everybody out eventually. You just can't stay in it. It catches up with everybody.
>
> *Researcher:* Was there any particular incident that triggered this?
>
> *Eric:* No, one day I was going great. March, a year ago I was doing just great. Next day I went to work, and I could hardly bring myself to face it. And nothing happened. It's not that I don't enjoy the work. I love helping people.

Several points stand out in this interview with Eric that may have a bearing on the phenomenon of burnout. First, Eric feels burned out but continues to work. Whatever his feelings are doing to him, he has not yet reached the point where he pursues another occupation. Second, despite his feeling that he is burned out, he still derives at least some satisfaction from his work. Something about the work still motivates him, and this seems to be his desire to be of help to others. Contrary to the findings of Maslach and Pines, some human-service workers may feel burned out, but not lose their concern for the clientele. And finally, in Eric's case, burnout did not come gradually. Without any particular incident or event, one day things were satisfactory, and the next day work could barely be faced. Obviously much more research needs to be done in this area to see if Eric's situation is unique. It is interesting that Eric cannot pinpoint in any precise way the beginnings of his troubles in terms of events, but he is fairly certain of the date when it all began. On that day in March he became aware of all that the work represented, particularly as it affected his own sense of mortality. He has come to the realization that maybe this work is for younger people, who without any obligations to wife and children or fears for their own self-preservation, are willing to confront and find reward in the many dangers and risks that accompany a career in emergency medicine.

CONCLUSION

In doing emergency ambulance work, EMTs and paramedics face stressful situations with which they must deal. Finding time and opportunity to eat, rest, and go to the bathroom, can be difficult achievements because the emergency runs on which they are sent follow no predictable pattern. Ambulance crews find that they must create their own opportunities of time and place to satisfy the basic physical necessities common to all human kind. Because emergency runs can occur at any moment, there is no way that EMTs and paramedics can "even out" the flow of their work. They frequently find themselves with time on their hands that must be filled in ways that are emotionally satisfying, but there are no formal or planned arrangements that can be made for filling the periods of waiting. Waiting periods are filled mostly with spontaneous activity such as shoptalk, games, and even doing errands. However, the underlying tension that any activity can be interrupted by a run is always there and pervades all time-out periods.

EMTs and paramedics also do risk-filled work; they are daily exposed to the hazards of high-speed city driving and the violence inherent in scenes of crime and domestic argument. The men and women who work in ambulance crews learn to live with risk and danger and accept it as part of their work. They lessen the stress that they feel by developing a relationship of interpersonal trust with their partner and other crew members; and developing an implicit faith in their own skills and in the safety and dependability of the vehicles they drive.

Theirs is also a world of death, trauma, and human tragedy in its most vivid and stark manifestations. They are exposed to the worst that illness and injury can impose on the unfortunate. Being human, EMTs and paramedics are sensitive to the suffering and anguish of the patients on whom they work. Yet they are mandated by the very nature of their chosen occupation to deliver the skills and techniques of emergency medicine in a way that is cool, calm, and competent, regardless of the human carnage that lies before them. EMTs and paramedics find that they can only do their work when they suppress their feelings and remain objective and detached. Because of this, however, opportunities must be created for the emotional component of their work to be given its proper due. The ambulance crews at County found that talking about what they had seen and done provided a necessary and helpful way of relieving their emotions. Colleagues, the company of fellow crew members, are those mostly readily sought for discussing a run, since only they can really understand what it meant to those involved.

With respect to burnout, for the older EMTs and paramedics, time begins to catch up. As the years roll by, the physical and emotional demands of the work take their toll. As Eric, the paramedic quoted earlier, and others of his age find out, their sense of mortality grabs hold, the work loses its excitement and stands over them and against them like a barrier—defying them to continue. And at a time when their medical wisdom is at its peak, their physical and emotional reserves are waning. Eric and others like him realize that they cannot continue much longer, but what work can they go to? If they have a degree and can teach or do administrative work, perhaps the classroom or the office desk can be their new setting. But if not, to what realms do they transfer their skills and special knowledge of the human condition that they have so arduously acquired?

Perhaps continuing education for EMTs and paramedics is very important. The more that is learned in the classroom through formal educational methods, the more that education can be transferred to other settings. But if we are to take at face value what EMTs and paramedics say, and which I myself have heard, most of what they must know to be of help to patients is "learned in the street," and how does such knowledge get transmitted and taught in the classroom? It is indeed a curious dilemma for the contemporary EMT and paramedic.

In the final analysis there are no perfect ways of coping with and adapting to the demands of emergency ambulance work. When EMTs and paramedics place an implicit trust in their driver, it does not lessen the risks that they take while driving; it only lessens their *feeling* of being in danger. But perhaps, after all, this is what really counts. Many years ago the sociologist W. I. Thomas asserted that if "men define a situation as real, it's real in its consequences."[21] This means that the EMTs and paramedics at County Hospital and elsewhere must and do create favorable definitions of their work if they are to work and have a career at all. They must find safety in danger, purpose while waiting, and most of all, some "good" in human illness and injury. They do indeed do this in their daily encounters with patients and colleagues as they attempt to render acceptable and make worthwhile the things that they face in their work.

8

THE FIELD EXPERIENCE

It was late in the afternoon, a warm, humid day in Metro-City, and I was sitting in the rear compartment of a paramedic ambulance. Dale was driving, and Eric, another paramedic was sitting in the back with me, examining some supplies in a cabinet. The dispatcher had given us a run for a personal-injury accident on one of the Metro-City expressways, and we were now heading down the entrance ramp preparing to merge into the heavy traffic.

We picked up more speed after we were onto the expressway, and I began nervously to check my seat belt to see if it would tighten a bit more. The noise became impressive, the roar of the motor, the loud wailing siren, the rattling of equipment, and the sound of the dispatcher's voice occasionally giving us more information about the location of the accident. I could tell that we were now traveling at a high speed as the cars we passed disappeared from view out the rear window.

I pictured in my mind what would happen if one of the drivers we were passing were to panic at the sound of our siren and suddenly steer over into our lane. I calculated that the impact at 80 or 90 miles per hour could kill us all. I gave a shudder and wondered to myself why I was there. I felt so vulnerable and unprotected. If I were to be severely injured in an accident doing this study— what would be the purpose? Would my university insurance cover it? Would it have been worthwhile? My mind was filled with these thoughts as I felt Dale accelerate still more. Was a field study of paramedics worth my getting hurt? I wanted it to be over. I wanted to be home or back at the hospital or in the crew room. To have my feet on the ground and to know I was safe. Again the thought returns to me—What am I doing here?[22]

I began this study of ambulance paramedics and EMTs in the summer of 1978, after spending a few months reviewing the literature, finding a research site, and gaining access to those persons whose permission and approval I would need to begin my research. As a medical sociologist, the field of emergency medical work held a certain fascination for me. A few years earlier my doctoral dissertation had focused on medical work in hospital emergency rooms. At that time my interests lay in the problems that emergency-room physicians and nurses face in carrying out their medical routines. I wanted to understand their world from their perspective, so I chose participant observation. The experience proved so satisfying to me intellectually, professionally, and personally that in 1978 I longed to return to the field and conduct another observational study. Emergency medicine was, and remains, a subject where good research is needed, and because not much had been published about emergency medicine in the prehospital setting, I felt that I could make a contribution. In particular, little was known in 1978 about emergency ambulance work from a sociological point of view, even though it was becoming increasingly evident through the popular media, medical journals, and other sources that emergency medical technicians and paramedics were doing some fairly important and sophisticated work, often with dramatic results. Ambulance technicians were no longer simply "first-aiders" or attendants; it appeared that ambulance work was no longer simply a transportation phenomenon. For these reasons and others I believed that this was something that needed research and that my past experience as an emergency-room observer would give me a sound basis for undertaking a field study of EMTs and paramedics.

In locating a research site, I decided that an urban medical system would be best since the volume of emergency cases would be greatest, and an urban area might be more likely to have a well-developed system of ambulance care, which would enhance the value of the research. Metro-City was known to me since I was an assistant professor at a small university in a community within commuting distance of it. Moreover, as a medical sociologist with interests in emergency medical work, I had heard of County Hospital's ambulance service, its paramedic program, and a little about its operations.

Through mutual friends I gained an interview with the director of emergency services at County Hospital. I told her of my interests and experiences as a researcher in the field of emergency medicine. I had drawn up a proposal for a field study of ambulance EMTs and paramedics, and I showed it to her. The director expressed enthusiasm for the study, and felt that as an observer, my insights into the world of ambulance workers might prove useful not only to me but also to them. However, final clearance for such a project had to come from the top of the hospital administration, and I was given an appointment with the County Hospital medical director. The medical director at the time of our interview had already examined my research proposal, and said that he had no problems with it, thought it might be of some value to the hospital, and that all that was needed now was final approval. I expected that would take a few weeks; it turned out to be a few months. I learned then, and had confirmed many times thereafer, that the administrative bureaucracies of hospitals such as County make decisions very carefully and slowly. Eventually permission was given to begin the study, and thereafter no problems were encountered. I am certain that my position as a professor at a nearby university of some reputation, as well as my previous research experience in hospital-emergency rooms, served to validate my status.

After waiting those months to begin field observation, I was now most anxious to start. The director of emergency medical services introduced me to two staff persons in the ambulance division. Both young men were involved in the daily operations of the division and were eager to learn about what I intended to study and how I expected to do it. I spent almost an entire day talking with them, getting insight into the routines of the ambulance service as well as suggestions about facets of EMT work that would be worth my observing. As an outsider I very much appreciated the goodwill and cooperation I received from these men and from the director of emergency medical services. I was told to feel free to make any observations I cared to make and to question anyone about anything I felt was important. There were absolutely no restrictions placed on my freedom of movement or lines of inquiry. Over the next eighteen months, I could not have asked for a more hospitable and cooperative group of people—from the top administrators to the ambulance EMTs. I never confronted antagonism, road blocks, or lack of cooperation. Virtually everything I asked for by way of information and assistance was willingly and openly given. Whatever problems I encountered in making observations—and there were some—were in no way related to the cooperation I sought and received from the ambulance division of County Hospital.

FIRST DAYS IN THE FIELD

In conducting the observations at County Hospital, I chose the role of the "known observer."[23] My decision was based on two considerations. First, in my previous research on hospital emergency rooms, I had played the same role and found it to be successful for my purposes. Second, without some degree of training, as an EMT for instance, there was really no other role I could play; I could not be an "unknown observer." I did not want to be an EMT, just so I could make observations, nor was it possible always to be at the scene as a bystander in making observations. So the role of known observer seemed necessary, but it also had many advantages. In doing participant observation, a known observer is more free to come and go as he or she pleases, and to ask questions about events and activities without fear of being discovered as an observer, or seeming more than a bit odd.

When field work was ready to begin one of the administrative staff of the ambulance division introduced me to Eric and Vince, two paramedics; explained to them the nature of the research I was doing; and told them I would be riding with them in their ambulance that day. We shook hands, and I climbed into the back of the ambulance and sat down.

My observational strategy called for me to observe first hand the daily work routines of the ambulance EMTs and paramedics at County. Since I could not observe all of them at once, I decided to ride and observe a crew for an entire shift of duty—reporting in when they did and ending at the close of the shift. Most of the observations were conducted with day-shift crews (7:00–3:00), although I did ride with several evening-shift crews (3:00–11:00). Once with a particular crew, I was required to stay with them at all times; since I wanted to accompany them on all their runs, I had to be nearby to hear communications from the dispatcher over the hand-held radio. While much of our time was spent in the ambulance, en route to the scene, or transporting to an emergency room, I also spent much time in the crew room, cafeterias, etc.—wherever the crew happened to go.

My most immediate problem in the beginning of the study was to establish and maintain rapport with the various crews with whom I was riding and observing. I was aided in these efforts by four important factors. First, the ambulance crews at County are accustomed to having observers ride with them. Doctors, nurses, and occasionally administrators have ridden as observers in an attempt to learn more about the street operations of the ambulance crews. Also student nurses and other EMTs in training ride as observers on a fairly regular basis. In this sense, the ambulance crews at County are used to having people looking over their shoulders. Second, my previous research on hospital emergency rooms had taught me how to be unobtrusive in medical emergencies. I knew how to observe without getting in the way. I will say more about this later. Third, I got the impression that many of the crews felt flattered that a sociologist was interested in their work, and they were eager to tell me about their world in the hope that what I observed would be written about so that others could better appreciate their work. Fourth, I was only slightly older than most of the EMTs and paramedics, and inasmuch as most of them were male, I had the advantage of whatever natural bonds exist among persons of the same age and sex. Also several of the EMTs and paramedics were college students or graduates, so that we shared some of the common cultural understandings of collegiate life.

Of the many different EMTs and paramedics at County I observed and talked to for more than a year and a half, I encountered no one who was antagonistic or uncooperative. On almost every occasion I was made to feel accepted and comfortable and I never sensed that I was in the way or a nuisance. This is not to say that all EMTs were equally easy to relate to. With some persons rapport was easily established, and little effort was required to have these persons share with me their feelings, attitudes, and values. With others, it took some work.

One example here should be illuminating. Alex, a black paramedic, was open with me, only if the other crew members were not around. As a black, Alex felt isolated—at the time of this study there were few black EMTs or paramedics—and between runs preferred to keep his own company. As long as I was willing to meet him on his terms, he would tell me about his work. I knew that the more time I spent alone with Alex, the more distant I became from the rest of the crew, but he had been working at County for some time, I felt it important that I get him to accept me. So he and I would sit alone in the ambulance between runs, while the rest of the crew would be enjoying the cameraderie of the crew room. In addition, Alex was a talker, and much of what he wanted to tell me was his philosophy of life or about experiences that had little to do with being a paramedic at County Hospital. To obtain the insights I was most interested in, I had to listen to a great deal of Alex's other thoughts. But I am a good listener and eventually my patience was rewarded.

Most of the paramedics and EMTs at County were not talkers at all, and while they would normally answer my questions, would not volunteer in any depth what they were not asked for. Moreover on some crews I felt that I was nothing much more than an observer, someone who was "there" for the day. On other crews I felt that I was accepted as something more; perhaps as someone they could not only trust but whom they rather enjoyed having around. I came to know many of them by their first names, and many knew me by mine. On several occasions I was invited to parties and to go "bar hopping" with a crew after the shift was over. I always declined these invitations as I am not good at drinking and driving.

Researchers in medical settings know that it is important that observational strategies not interfere with the work being conducted. No doubt, many observers have suffered the embarrassment of a doctor or nurse having to tell them to "get out of the way" or "leave the room" or "save your question for later, I'm busy!" After all critical work is often being conducted, and an overly inquisitive observer can at times only add to the confusion of the scene. I knew this to be especially true in medical emergencies, and knew also that one of the ways I could gain acceptance as a researcher was to stay out of the way in a "sticky" situation and save my questions for a more opportune time. Following this simple rule, there were no occasions when I felt my presence was a hindrance, nor was I asked to remove myself from the scene. I came to learn that after the emergency victim was transported to the hospital, the crew normally spent some time discussing the run while they cleaned out the ambulance or returned to County—and these occasions provided ample opportunity for asking questions and holding informal interviews.

INFORMANTS

In the strictest sense of the word, I did not recruit or use any informants. There were several paramedics whom I got along with very well, and I relied on them more than others to answer some of my questions and to get their point of view. In addition, one paramedic, a veteran of several years at County, agreed to some in-depth, taped interviews, which I conducted toward the end of the field-observation phase. These taped interviews were held to verify, from the perspective of a highly experienced paramedic, some of the observations I was making. In short, I wanted to know how close my interpretation was to the paramedic point of view. In other words, was I on the right track or not?

It was my good fortune that this paramedic was not only articulate and agreeable, but a person whose powers of observation and interpretation were the equal of many a social scientist. I am very gratified he was willing to share them with me.

BEING OF HELP

Field researchers often find that they are called upon to be of help to those they are observing in return for the cooperation they seek. To the degree that the observer agrees to be of help, he or she often gains a sense of trust and rapport as others come to accept more fully someone who is willing to assist them. Eliot Liebow found, for example, in his study of black street-corner men that his willingness to do important things for some of the street-corner men gave him crucial validation as a white man who could be counted on.[24] As I was not an EMT or paramedic, there were not many ways in which I could be of help to the crews I was observing. Yet there were opportunities for me to show that I could be useful, which enhanced my credibility. At an emergency scene I would often assist in getting the stretcher-cot from the ambulance or fetch some supplies or piece of equipment that was needed. On other occasions I would hold a bag of IV solution, or help lift a patient onto the stretcher-cot. As an observer, I always had plenty of notebooks and pens with me and loaned them out when needed. None of the services that I performed were necessarily dramatic or crucial, but they served to establish that I could be counted on—and what is probably more important showed that I was not afraid to roll up my sleeves and get my hands dirty.

PERSONAL FEELINGS

Every field researcher develops personal feelings and attitudes about the setting he or she is observing and the participants who constitute the subject matter. I doubt that any observer would choose to study a setting or group of people that he or she abhorred. If a sociologist felt homosexuality was repugnant, it would take an almost heroic fortitude for that researcher to do field work in gay baths, for example. On the other hand, our understanding of social settings and participants will never be advanced if researchers study only what they find naturally agreeable or acceptable.

In studying medical work in emergency contexts, it is difficult to think of the study or setting in negative terms. Few would disagree with the statement that the work that ambulance crews do is sometimes repugnant but never unworthy—maybe unpleasant but not unimportant. As a researcher, it was difficult for me not to be sympathetic toward the ambulance crews I was observing. Much of their work was performed at considerable risk and danger to their own personal safety. During the study several EMTs and paramedics were seriously injured in collisions en route to emergency scenes. They performed their work in all sorts of inclement weather—in the cold, the heat, the dark. They treated anyone in any condition who requested their help; and they daily witnessed the tragedies of the human condition—death, traumatic injuries, child abuse, etc. For all this, they did not get paid a great deal of money, and only on some occasions were they able to save and prolong human life.

Indeed, in light of the above, I found that my natural sympathies must not be allowed to interfere with my objectivity as a researcher. Here was a group of men and women who, with few exceptions, brought a sense of commitment and dignity to their work, despite their relatively limited training and fairly low placement in the hierarchy of American medical care. In fact, for some of the population, these are merely ambulance attendants. The aim of my research though was not to paint a sympathetic view of emergency ambulance crews so that the public would better appreciate this kind of work. My purpose was to see their work and the many problems associated with that work from their point of view. It was to gain a sense of their perspective on their world. While some of what I have written is flattering, no doubt; some of it is just the opposite. I tried to avoid seduction; I talked to everyone who would talk to me; and attempted insofar as possible, to render faithfully and objectively what was seen and heard.

I found that my lot as a researcher was to be the plight of any and all field observers—to be in the setting but not of it. I was there, physically present as a sociologist, and accepted as a person who deserved to be there. I was "the sociologist." Sometimes at the scene of an automobile accident, for example, a policeman might ask one of the crew, "Who is this guy?" pointing at me. The paramedic would answer, "He's with us. He's trying to figure us out for a study he's doing." That was my role, "to figure them out for a study," and it was a lonely pursuit to be there as observer and analyst, almost as though I were not an actual person at all.

There were further difficulties. On the one hand, although observations are relatively easy to make, the analysis of them is not. You can see what is going on before your eyes, who is doing and saying what to whom; but what it all means and where it fits in the larger scheme of things is another matter. When an observer tries to observe and analyze at the same time, it takes a great deal of continuous thought and energy. It means being alert and attentive at all times. When a crew took some time out in the crew room to relax between runs, I could not afford the luxury. Often what was said and done in the crew room was critical to my research. That is where many of the values and attitudes about EMT work were shared and discussed. No matter how much I might have wanted to remove myself to my private thoughts and dreams, I had to be just as observant and alert to conversation and behavior there as I was in the street at the scene of an emergency. For me, there were no time-outs. Almost everything said was grist for my sociological mill. I found that at the end of an eight-hour shift I was quite exhausted.

This leads me to expand upon a point mentioned earlier. On more than one occasion I was invited to attend a party held at the home of one of the ambulance workers. These were ambulance division parties in the sense that all the County EMTs and paramedics were invited and most would attend. I never accepted these invitations because I was never sure what my role at the party should be. If I did not go, it would give the others an opportunity to talk about the sociologist and air their feelings. This they would be unlikely to do should I be present. More-over, if I did attend, and the EMTs and paramedics decided to talk shop and discuss runs and compare notes on cases, could I—and indeed should I—resist the temptation to play the role of researcher and use the material gathered there for my study? It would be a superb oppor-tunity, but would it be fair for me as an invited guest to do so? After all, work was over. And if the guests suspected I was there as an ob-server, would they feel free to have fun and say what they wanted to in the presence of the sociologist? To me, the complications were mani-fold. As a researcher I had to be marginal, a researcher of work behavior but not one close enough to be an invited guest at a party. I did not want to be "of" the group for fear that the emotional involvements might compromise me.

COLLECTING THE DATA

The period of observations for this study spanned eighteen months. My field observations began in the summer of 1978 and continued through the fall of 1979. During the summer months I used my vacation time to ride as an observer several days a week. When college was in session, and I had pressing academic obligations, I would go into the field only once or twice a week. As stated earlier, I would ride for an entire eight-hour shift of duty with one crew, and since the crews rotated around the different stations in Metro-City, I eventually rode with nearly all the crews. In all a total of some five hundred hours of direct field observations were conducted.

In addition to the direct observations I held informal and semistructured interviews with many County EMTs and paramedics. And, as stated earlier, with one paramedic I conducted several hours of structured in-depth interviews. This person was chosen for in-depth interviewing because he had worked at County for many years and could give me historical perspective on the developments of the EMT and paramedic program. He was an articulate person who had done a lot of reflecting about ambulance work. Furthermore, he was interested in the study and wanted to make a contribution of some sort. The other semistructured and unstructured interviews were held with those who were the most talkative and the most willing to open up to me. Usually these interviews consisted of informal question-and-answer periods held in the crew room between runs or while we were having lunch or sitting in the back of an ambulance resting. Since the dispatch operation is vital to County's emergency response system, I also spent some shifts sitting in Control observing the work of the dispatchers.

The decision about when to observe—that is to say, what particular shifts to observe—was largely made as a matter of convenience. Travel considerations made the day-shift crews more convenient to observe. Evening-shift crews have a heavier volume of emergency runs because of increased traffic flow, children home from school, and so forth, so I made it a point to observe during the evening shifts as well.

NOTE TAKING

When I am in the field, I prefer not to take a lot of notes in the presence of participants. I have the feeling that it bothers people to see someone writing down everything they say. On the other hand, if you are to play the role of observer, there are times when participants, no doubt, expect the researcher to take some notes to show that he or she is working and is taking the study seriously. Quite aside from this, I found it very difficult to take notes riding in an ambulance. The bumping and swaying of the vehicle permitted only the sketchiest attempts.

I decided to carry with me in the field several small notebooks in which I could record short notes and conversations. Through the years

I have developed my own shorthand, which is understood only by me, but is a convenient and effective way of taking notes while on the run. During time-out periods in the crew room, while at lunch, or relaxing in the back of the ambulance, I would jot notes into my several notebooks. These would be bits and pieces of conversations, phrases to remind me of certain events. Even analytical categories might be jotted down if important ideas occurred to me in the field.

At the end of the shift, I would remain at the hospital for several hours writing up fuller field notes. In my briefcase I would have several larger notebooks, and in the professional library of County Hospital I would take my jottings and develop them into full field notes, while events and conversations were still fresh in my memory.

My home was over an hour's drive from Metro-City, and upon reaching there I would tape-record all the day's jotted and full field notes, plus any other items concerning the observations that had occurred to me on the journey home. I found that the hour's drive was useful for reflecting and sorting out that day's or evening's activities, and many useful ideas for analysis came to me during this period.

Once all the notes were recorded, I had two records of observations: the tapes and the field notes from the hospital. From the tapes I would search for categories and lines of analysis, a process that I will describe shortly.

In addition to these materials I also gathered other kinds of data important to the study. All kinds of printed material pertaining to the operations of the ambulance crews were collected. Run sheets, administrative directives to the EMTs, office bulletins, were the sorts of secondary materials that could provide useful insights into the daily work routine. I also carefully perused the Metro-City newspapers for accounts of emergencies involving ambulance crews from County Hospital. I kept a separate file on all this material. In addition, I made certain to watch the television coverage of emergency scenes in Metro-City, especially of those involving EMT and paramedic crews. When possible, I would take notes on the television coverage, seeing, for example, if I could identify some or all of the crews by name. Of course, since the television news coverage of emergency events involves taping for the late evening news show, I was often able to see myself playing the role of observer at an important Metro-City emergency.

DIFFICULT OBSERVATIONS

I am certain every observer finds that in the course of a field study some events are easier to witness and record than others; either because they are less unpleasant, less fearful, or whatever. As an observer of emergency ambulance crews, I had to see and confront all that they did, and much of it required a strong stomach and a sense of fortitude. My work in hospital emergency rooms had prepared me for some of it, but there is something about witnessing emergency events "in the street" that makes them much more stark.

As we saw earlier, paramedics and EMTs get used to working on people who are dead, dying, mutilated, and suffering. And in time I got used to it too. But at first it was difficult for me. I do not like the sight of blood, the sounds that people in great pain make, the sight of broken limbs and mangled bodies. I remember one event early in the field study in which the paramedic crew I was observing was called to meet a township ambulance en route to Mercy Hospital. We learned from the dispatcher that an eight-year-old girl had been run over by a truck. When we met the other ambulance, Vince and Terry, the paramedics I was with, quickly climbed into the other ambulance and beckoned me to join them. I could not face it at first. I did not want to see what the child might look like, and I devoutly wished that I had never begun the field study. I did not want to be there; I just could not do it. However, I took some deep breaths and told myself that this is what the study was about: how men and women trained as EMTs and paramedics manage medical emergencies. This was an event that I had to witness not only because it was an important piece of data for the study but also because I had to maintain my credibility with the crew. What would they think of me as a researcher if I could not really observe them in action as I had said I would? So I found the fortitude to enter the ambulance, saw Vince cutting away with scissors the young girl's clothing, saw a leg bone obviously badly fractured, a large crushing injury on the head, and watched as Vince and Terry calmly started IV lines and talked by two-way radio to a physician at Mercy Hospital. I made the observation, but those runs where people were dying and severely injured and mutilated never became any easier. The nights afterward I never slept well, staring at the ceiling and wondering what had happened to those so badly hurt or gravely ill.

Here I have touched on a problem faced by researchers of emergency medical scenes. When emergency ambulance workers face patients in great distress, part of the way in which they are able to cope or deal with it is to do the work they were trained to do. They apply the skills and techniques of their occupation and hope for a successful outcome. In a sense, this is what they are there for. I as a researcher was there to record events and activities, and there is not much I could attempt to do for the patient. In that regard, I was helpless. About the only consolation I had was that perhaps the insights produced from my study would be of help to someone, sometime, somewhere. But that would indeed be in the long run. In the meantime I could only stand and observe and faithfully record.

ANALYSIS

My original purpose in undertaking this study was to write one or two articles on how ambulance paramedics and EMTs manage to cope with the various medical emergencies they confront. As my field work continued, I came to realize that it was difficult to describe the complexities of this kind of medical work in a single article. Eventually, as I began to search for the meaningful categories in which to arrange the data, a much larger manuscript began to unfold. One line of inquiry led to another until I began to realize that many of these categories were closely linked and the parts could not be understood without understanding the whole.

To return once again briefly to my method of procedure, because it is relevant to this discussion, after I had taped all the field notes, I would transcribe from the tapes the notes and search for categories. Some of the notes fitted more than one analytic category, and when they did I cross-referrenced them. I put the notes on 5″ by 7″ cards, numbered them and alphabetized them and filed them in large filing boxes. This was the basic technique for recording and retrieving the data.

My perspective from the beginning never really shifted, it only expanded. The focus was always on how human beings confront the problematic aspects of their daily work, render it meaningful and sensible, and cope with and adapt to those problematic features. And since a sociological perspective was used, I concentrated on the shared, collective strategies EMTs and paramedics employed in coping with their world.

In addition, I also wanted to do a treatise on the work. What was it like to do this sort of emergency medical work, or as Hughes put it, to perform routinely what for others were emergency events? How the work is carried out and made routine became an important theme.

From the beginning to the end of the study I had in mind presenting as much of the data as I could from the perspective of the men and women who performed the work. To see their world on their terms, using their categories of reality and definition. Admittedly some of the subcategories used in the body of the data analysis were "observer-generated," but many more were "participant-generated."

While the original focus did not shift dramatically, it did expand, and this transformed an article into a book-length manuscript. A few examples may be helpful here. At the outset I wanted to study only paramedics—or those EMTs with advanced training who do ambulance work. I soon discovered, however, that virtually all paramedics come up from EMT ranks, and although the work of the paramedic is more sophisticated and advanced, the orientation of the EMT and paramedic toward work, medicine, and patients is very much alike. Therefore since many EMTs also eventually become paramedics, I did not focus exclusively on paramedics and included EMTs in my interviews and observations.

In addition, my original plans called for me to concentrate heavily on paramedic conduct during acute medical emergencies. Here again, I soon came to realize that not all the runs EMTs and paramedics respond to are of an acute nature. As we saw in Chapter 5, not all runs are for what almost anyone could call an emergency. EMTs and paramedics also spend a great deal of time waiting for something to happen. If I were to focus only on the acute emergencies, I would be a long time gathering data. On some shifts I might be able to observe several such runs; on others I might not see one. Consequently, I decided that I would look at the entire daily routine of EMTs and paramedics. As it turned out, I believe that this was a wise decision. One of the most important features of doing EMT work is learning to balance the demands of an acute medical emergency with the less serious one, and finding some sense of satisfaction in the intervals of waiting for something to happen. To be a paramedic or EMT, one cannot live only for the emergency runs; one must also learn to find enjoyment in the company of equals in the crew room or wherever the periods of waiting are spent.

LOOKING BACK

Every research experience is filled with moments of triumph as well as times of trial and tribulation. It seems to be true, however, that probably the biggest mistakes or shortcomings in field observations are never discovered. There remains always the nagging suspicion that important items were overlooked, that key persons were never talked to, that trivial matters were magnified and significant ones given only brief mention. Time will provide an answer to these questions, and it is not up to me to decide the issue. Certainly observations in the field of emergency ambulance crews are not always easy to make, especially during a medical emergency. So many things happen at once. Someone is attending to the patient; others are obtaining information from relatives and bystanders. Policemen and perhaps firemen are scurrying about. Perhaps one of the paramedics is talking to a physician by two-way radio. Which action or persons are most important? To concentrate on one element is to miss others, and maybe what is missed turns out to be the most important. An observer cannot be everywhere at once, and he or she must be selective. But on what grounds do you decide what and whom you observe? This is a question not easily answered. Here is one example of the dilemma.

When a paramedic unit was to transport a patient to an emergency facility, I had my choice as to where I would ride en route. Should I ride in the rear compartment with the paramedics and the patient, or should I ride in front with the EMT driver? If I rode in the front, the EMT was free to talk because he or she was driving and was not occupied in taking care of the patient. I could ask questions about the run, how the decision when to transport was made, what this run meant in relation to other runs that day, and so on. If the EMT driver was open and responsive, I could obtain a good deal of information about the run. However, I could not know what was going on in the rear compartment unless I left my seat and crawled back there. If I chose to ride in the rear compartment, I would see at first hand what was being done to and for the patient, and I would hear the paramedics exchanging information. But since the paramedics would be occupied with the patient, I could not question them until we arrived at the emergency room and the patient was admitted. If we were called on another run shortly thereafter, I might not have the time or opportunity to get background information about the run, in terms of the values and attitudes involved. So on every transport I had to choose, and of course, I tried to even up the number of times I rode in the back and up front. The only problem was that when I rode in the rear, I felt that I would have gained more by talking to the driver, and when I rode in front, my mind wondered what was taking place behind my back.

Did my presence as an observer made a difference in how the EMTs and paramedics conducted themselves? No doubt, it did to a degree, but I can only hope that in general what I saw and described would hold up with another observer. As mentioned earlier, EMTs are used to having people around. At an emergency scene there are all kinds of people watching them work, so that the presence of a sociologist is probably not all that significant.

I close this chapter and book by revealing one haunting aspect of the nature of my research in medical emergency work. Because I was interested in making observations on ambulance EMTs and paramedics as they performed their duties and managed medical emergencies, it meant that I had to see them in action. From the EMT and paramedic standpoint, they too want action—a "good run," as we have seen, being one in which they can utilize their medical skills and abilities. All of us, observer and participants, spent a good deal of time waiting for these emergency events to occur, and I found myself more and more adopting their perspective and point of view. When it was a slow shift, the ambulance crew anxiously awaited the dispatcher's call for what would hopefully prove to be a good run. As an observer, I too was awaiting a run in which the medical judgments were critical and I could observe at first hand how they were made and the emergency managed.

As a result, I began to have some misgivings about my role, because like the EMTs and paramedics other people's misfortune and tragedy were my awaited work. But unlike the paramedics, who were bringing help to the victim and making routine what others considered dangerous emergency work, What was I doing besides collecting information? My interesting observational data, vignettes, and examples of emergency medical work on the dying or the traumatically injured were gathered at someone else's extraordinary expense. In order for someone to do this work, whether paramedic or sociologist-observer, others had to have a coronary, an accident, swallow poison, run over a child, or commit suicide. In this year and a half of my life, I shared with these emergency workers the irony of all who earn their living from other people's tragedies, doctors and nurses included. For me the irony is still greater and more haunting since I brought no medical help to the side of the patient. This is part of the very solitary life of the medical observer, to be willing to observe but unable to help. To those whose medical misfortunes made possible the data, my work, and this study, please know that in my own way I shared in your sorrows.

REFERENCES

Throughout the writing of this book I was aided significantly by the following two studies:

Douglas, D., "Occupational and Therapeutic Contingencies of Ambulance Services in Metropolitan Areas," Ph.D. dissertation, University of California, 1969.

Rubinstein, J., *City Police*. New York: Random House, 1973.

For those readers interested in learning more about occupational burnout, I found the following articles very helpful:

Maslach, C., and Jackson, M., "Burned-out Cops and Their Families." *Psychology Today,* May, 59–62, 1979.

Maslach, C., "Burned-out." *Human Behavior,* 5, 16–22, 1975.

Freudenberger, H., "Staff Burnout." *Journal of Social Issues,* 30, 159–165, 1974.

1.　Fox, R., *Experiment Perilous* (Glencoe: Free Press, 1959); and Freidson, E., *The Profession of Medicine* (New York: Dodd, Mead, & Co., 1970).
2.　Merton, R., Reader, G., and Kendall, P., eds., *The Student Physician* (Cambridge: Harvard University Press, 1957).
3.　Mannon, J., "Defining and Treating Problem Patients in a Hospital Emergency Room." *Medical Care,* 14, 12, 1004–1013, 1976.
4.　Scheff, T., "Decision Rules, Types of Error and Consequences for Medical Diagnosis." *Behavioral Science,* 8, 97–107, 1963.
5.　Freidson, E., *The Profession of Medicine* (New York: Dodd, Mead & Co., 1970).
6.　See Sudnow, D., *Passing On* (Englewood Cliffs: Prentice-Hall, 1967), p. 127.
7.　Davis, F., *Passage Through Crisis* (Indianapolis: Bobbs-Merrill, 1963).
8.　Giffin, K., "Interaction Variables of Interpersonal Trust." *Humanities,* 9, 297–315, 1973.
9.　Hughes, E. C., *The Sociological Eye,* Vol. II (New York: Aldine-Atherton, 1971).
10.　– – –, *The Sociological Eye,* p. 343.

11. Becker, H., Geer, B., Hughes, E., Straus. *Boys in White* (Chicago: University of Chicago Press, 1961).

12. Roth, J., "Some Contingencies of the Moral Evaluation and Control of Clientele." *American Journal of Sociology,* 77, 839–856, 1972.

13. See for example Goode, W., "Community Within a Community: The Professions." *American Sociological Review,* 194–200, 1957; Parsons, T., "The Professions as Social Structure," in *Essays in Sociological Theory,* 34–47 (New York: Free Press, 1954); Greenwood, E., "Attributes of a Profession." *Social Work* II, July, 45–55, 1957.

14. Krause, E., *Power and Illness* (New York: Elsevier, 1977).

15. Dutten, L., Smolensky, M., Lorimor, R., Hsi, B., Leach, G., "Psychological Stress Levels in Paramedics." *Emergency Medical Services,* 88–94, September/ October, 1978.

16. Haas, J., "Learning Real Feelings: A Study of High Steel Ironworkers' Reactions to Fear and Danger." *Sociology of Work and Occupations,* 14, 12, 147–70, 1977.

17. See for example Coombes, R., and Goldman, L., "Maintenance and Discontinuity of Coping Mechanisms in an Intensive Care Unit," *Social Problems,* 20, 342–355, 1973.

18. Freudenberger, H., "Staff Burn-out." *Journal of Social Issues,* 30, 159–165, 1974.

19. Maslach, C., Pines, A., "The Burn-out Syndrome in the Day Care Setting." *Child Care Quarterly,* 6, 100–113, 1977.

20. McSwain, N., Shelton, M., "Burnout—Real or Imagined?" *Topics in Emergency Medicine,* 1, 4, 93–97, 1980.

21. Thomas, W. I., *The Child in America* (New York: Knopf, 1928), p. 572.

22. This chapter is based on a format presented in Lofland, J., *Analyzing Social Settings* (Belmont: Wadsworth, 1971).

23. Gold, R., "Roles in Sociological Field Observations." *Social Forces,* 36, 217–223, 1958.

24. Liebow, E., *Tally's Corner* (Boston: Little, Brown, 1967).

INDEX